100 Uplifting

Short Stories

for Seniors

© Copyright 2024 - All rights reserved.

You may not reproduce, duplicate or send the contents of this book without direct written permission from the author. You cannot hereby despite any circumstance blame the publisher or hold him or her to legal responsibility for any reparation, compensations, or monetary forfeiture owing to the information included herein, either in a direct or an indirect way.

Legal Notice: This book has copyright protection. You can use the book for personal purposes. You should not sell, use, alter, distribute, quote, take excerpts, or paraphrase in part or whole the material contained in this book without obtaining the permission of the author first.

Disclaimer Notice: You must take note that the information in this document is for casual reading and entertainment purposes only. We have made every attempt to provide accurate, up-to-date, and reliable information. We do not express or imply guarantees of any kind. The persons who read admit that the writer is not occupied in giving legal, financial, medical, or other advice. We put this book content by sourcing various places.

Please consult a licensed professional before you try any techniques shown in this book. By going through this document, the book lover comes to an agreement that under no situation is the author accountable for any forfeiture, direct or indirect, which they may incur because of the use of material contained in this document, including, but not limited to, a errors, omissions, or inaccuracies.

Introduction

Welcome to "100 Uplifting Short Stories for Seniors" — a delightful journey through decades of laughter, nostalgia, and genuine human experiences. In this charming collection, you'll find a treasure trove of funny and heartwarming tales that are sure to bring a smile to your face and warmth to your heart.

Each story in this book is crafted with care and attention to detail, drawing inspiration from real-life events and experiences. While the stories may be written with humor and wit, they are firmly rooted in truth, offering readers a glimpse into the quirks and joys of everyday life.

As you turn the pages of this book, you'll meet a colorful cast of characters and embark on a series of adventures that will leave you laughing, reminiscing, and maybe even shedding a tear or two. From humorous mishaps to heartwarming moments of connection, these stories capture the essence of what it means to be human — flawed, funny, and infinitely resilient.

So, sit back, relax, and prepare to be entertained. Whether you're reading alone or sharing these stories with loved ones, "100 Uplifting Short Stories for Seniors" is sure to brighten your day and remind you of the simple joys that make life worth living. Enjoy the journey, and may these stories bring a little extra sunshine into your world.

Table of Contents
- Introduction 3

LET'S GO BACK TO THE 50'S 7
- The Great Ice Cream Caper 8
- The Quirky Quack-Up: The Case of the Dancing Duck 10
- The Chicken Who Laid Square Eggs 12
- The Great TP Tango: A Tale of Toilet Paper Panic 15
- Briefs in Bloom: The Great Underwear Hoax 17
- Gone in a Flash: The Mystery of the Vanishing Car 19
- The Canine Comedian: The Tale of the Talking Dog 22
- The Case of the Missing Pie: A Sweet Mystery Unraveled 24
- The Alien Antics: A Close Encounter of the Mischief Kind 26
- Trunk Trouble: The Tale of the Escaped Circus Elephant 28
- The Mischievous Monkey Mischief: A Whimsical Tale of an Escaped Primate 30
- The Out-of-This-World Prank: A Whimsical Tale of the Great "Flying Saucer" Hoax 31
- The Clucking Conundrum: A Feathered Tale of the Mystery of the Dancing Chicken 33
- The Tail of the Three-Legged Cat: A Whimsical Tale of Feline Frolics 34
- The Invisible Dog Debacle: A Hilarious Tale of Imaginary Antics 36
- The Pie-Eating Fiasco: A Legendary Tale of Culinary Chaos 37
- The Quacking Canine Companion: A Tail-Wagging Tale of Unlikely Friendship 39
- The Sock Puppet Spectacle: An Unforgettable Tale of Whimsy and Wonder 40
- The Great Toilet Paper Caper: A Tale of Comical Chaos 42
- The Hilarious Hijinks of the Amateur Talent Show 43

LET'S GO BACK TO THE 60'S 45
- The Bikini Bust: A Tale of the Great Swimsuit Ban 46
- Fab Four Fiasco: The Beatles' Pillow Fight Frenzy 48
- Dolly Doppelgängers: The Hilarious Tale of the Look-Alike Contest 50
- Mice in Space: The Hilarious Tale of NASA's Great Mouse Invasion 52
- The Sock Rebellion: A Hilarious Tale of the Great Sock Protest 54
- The Stinky Showdown: A Whiffy Tale of the Smelliest Football Game 56
- Flamingo Fiasco: The Hilarious Tale of the Great Stolen Lawn Flamingo Caper 58
- The Paw-litical Candidate: A Tail of the Poodle Who Ran for Mayor 60
- The Elevator Escapade: A Hilarious Tale of the Great Stuck Elevator Incident 62
- The Sticky Situation: A Whimsical Tale of the Great Bubble Gum Wall Incident 64
- The Twisted Tango: A Hilarious Tale of the Great "Twist" Dance-Off 66
- Woof Couture: The Whimsical Tale of the Space-Age Dog Fashion Show 68
- The Peanut Prank Pandemonium: A Nutty Tale That Had the Whole Campus Cracking Up 70
- Disco Duck Mania: A Quacky Tale of the Great "Disco Duck" Craze 72
- The Hot Dog Havoc: A Hilarious Tale of the Epic Eating Contest Mishap 74

The Melodic Mischief of the Singing Goldfish: A Fishy Tale 76
The Rubber Chicken Riot: A Feather-Ruffling Fiasco 78
The Lively Llama Limousine Adventure: A Tale of Llamas and Laughter 80
The Hilarious Horseplay: A Tale of the Pantomime Horse Parade Prank 82
Granny's Groovy Glide: The Tale of the Unexpected Skateboarding Granny 84

LET'S GO BACK TO THE 70'S 86

The Rock Stars: A Rockin' Tale of the Great Pet Rock Craze 87
The Disco Debacle: A Hilarious Tale of the "Disco Sucks" Rally 89
The Fizzy Fiasco: A Comical Tale of the Infamous "Coke" Hoax 91
The Grinning Epidemic: A Whimsical Tale of the Great "Smile Face" Craze 92
The Wacky Races: A Zany Tale of Legendary Laughter 94
The Bovine Bungle: A Moo-ving Tale of the Case of the Stolen Cow Mascot 96
The Sweet Shambles: A Whimsical Tale of The Great "Candy Necklace" Incident 98
The Clucking Comedy: A Feather-Ruffling Tale of The "Funky Chicken" Dance-Off 100
The Peculiar Poodle Puzzle: A Hilarious Tale of the Missing "Poodle" 101
The Leisure Suit Lunacy: A Silly Tale of the Great "Leisure Suit" Fad 103
Disco Demolition Delirium: A Comical Tale of "Disco Demolition" Night 104
The Doughnut Dilemma: A Whimsical Tale of the Missing Giant Doughnut 106
The Rubber Chicken Revelry: A Hilarious Tale of the Great "Rubber Chicken" Parade 108
The Cheeky Craze: A Whimsical Tale of the "Mooning" Fad 110
The Silly String Showdown: A Wacky Tale of the Great "Silly String" War 112
The Sign Snafu: A Whimsical Tale of the Stolen Street Sign 113
The Toga Tumult: A Comical Tale of The Great "Toga Party" Escapade 115
The Gorilla-Suit Guffaw: A Whimsical Tale of The Missing Gorilla Suit 116
The Whoopee Cushion Caper: A Hilarious Tale of The Prank Gone Pffft! 118
The Watery Wobble: A Splashy Tale of The Great "Waterbed" Fad 119

LET'S GO BACK TO THE 80'S 121

The Cabbage Caper: A Zany Tale of The Great Cabbage Patch Kids Craze 122
The Mullet Mayhem: A Hairy Tale of The Rise of the Mullets 123
The Cola Catastrophe: A Fizzy Tale of The Infamous "New Coke" Debacle 125
The Pac-Man Pandemonium: A Retro Tale of the "Pac-Man Fever" Phenomenon 126
The Fashion Fiasco: A Hilarious Tale of Outrageous Fashion Trends 128
The Cube Craze: A Whimsical Tale of Rubik's Cube Mania 129
The Walkman Whimsy: A Comical Tale of the Sony Walkman Introduction 131
The Aerobics Antics: A Laugh-Out-Loud Tale of Hilarious Workout Videos 132
The Hair-Raising Hilarity: A Rockin' Tale of Hair Metal Bands 134
The Silly Sayings Saga: A Chuckle-Worthy Tale of The "Just Say No" Campaign 135
The Zany Zeal of "Weird Al": A Whimsical Tale of Popularity 137
The Groovy Ghoul Gala: A Spooky Tale of The Thriller Dance Craze 138

THE PUNK ROCK PANDEMONIUM: A RIOTOUS TALE OF REBELLION 140
THE SILLY SATURDAY SHENANIGANS: A WHIMSICAL TALE OF SATURDAY MORNING CARTOONS 141
THE DISMAL DELOREAN DISASTER: A HILARIOUS TALE OF EPIC FAIL 143
THE VHS VENDETTA: A HILARIOUS TALE OF VIDEO RENTAL STORE INVASION... 144
THE BEEFY BLUNDER: A CHUCKLE-INDUCING TALE OF THE "WHERE'S THE BEEF?" CATCHPHRASE 146
THE HAIR-RAISING HARMONIES: A HILARIOUS TALE OF HAIR BANDS' BALLADS 147
THE COMICAL CONUNDRUM OF EARLY COMPUTERS: A LAUGHABLE TALE OF TECHNOLOGICAL AWKWARDNESS 149
THE MIAMI VICE FASHION FIASCO: A RIOTOUS TALE OF OUTRAGEOUSNESS 150

LET'S GO BACK TO THE 90'S 152

THE BEANIE BABY BONANZA: A WHIMSICAL TALE OF FURRY FRENZY.. 153
THE MACARENA MAYHEM: A HILARIOUS TALE OF DANCEFLOOR DELIRIUM 154
THE TAMAGOTCHI TUMULT: A COMICAL TALE OF DIGITAL PET PANDEMONIUM 156
THE BOY BAND BOOM: A CHEEKY TALE OF CROONING CHARM 157
THE FRESH PRINCE FIASCO: A ZANY TALE OF SITCOM SHENANIGANS 159
THE POKÉMON PANDEMONIUM: A WACKY TALE OF POCKET MONSTERS 160
THE CYBER CAFE CRAZE: A HILARIOUS TALE OF ONLINE ODYSSEY 162
THE Y2K YIKES: A LAUGHABLE TALE OF MILLENNIUM MAYHEM 163
THE FANNY PACK FIASCO: A RIDICULOUS TALE OF FASHION FAUX PAS... 165
THE FRIENDS FIASCO: A HILARIOUS TALE OF SITCOM SHENANIGANS.. 166
THE SAVED BY THE BELL SHENANIGANS: A ZANY TALE OF TEENAGE TURMOIL... 168
THE BAYWATCH BROUHAHA: A BEACHY TALE OF BIZARRE LIFEGUARDING... 169
THE POG PANDEMONIUM: A WACKY TALE OF SLAMMER SLAPSTICK... 171
THE AIM ANTICS: A HILARIOUS TALE OF DIGITAL DIALOGUE 172
THE TWIN PEAKS WHIRLWIND: A ZANY TALE OF SMALL-TOWN MYSTERY 174
THE GRUNGE FASHION FRENZY: A WACKY TALE OF FLANNEL AND DOC MARTENS 175
THE SIMPSONS SHENANIGANS: A ZANY TALE OF YELLOW FAMILY HIJINKS... 177
THE O.J. SIMPSON SAGA: A QUIRKY TALE OF COURTROOM CAPERS 178
THE DIAL-UP DELIGHT: A HILARIOUS JOURNEY INTO THE WORLD WIDE WEB 180
THE SEINFELD SAGA: A HILARIOUS ROMP THROUGH SITCOM SHENANIGANS... 181

Let's go Back

To the 50's

The Great Ice Cream Caper

In the sweltering summer of 1956, the small town of Sunnyvale was hit with a wave of mischief that would go down in history as The Great Ice Cream Caper. It all started innocently enough, with the cheerful jingle of the ice cream truck echoing through the neighborhood streets like a siren call to children far and wide.

Little did the ice cream truck driver know, he was about to become the unwitting star of a slow-speed chase that would have the whole town talking for years to come.

As the truck trundled down Main Street, its colorful exterior adorned with pictures of tempting treats, a group of mischievous kids hatched a plan that would go down in infamy. With a twinkle in their eyes and mischief in their hearts, they leaped into action.

First, they scattered like ants at a picnic, each child strategically positioning themselves at different points along the route, ready to pounce at the perfect moment. Then, as the ice cream truck slowed to a stop at its usual spot by the park, the ringleader of the group, young Timmy, made his move.

With the precision of a seasoned criminal mastermind (or so he liked to think), Timmy darted forward and, quicker than a rabbit in a carrot patch, clambered into the driver's seat of the unattended ice cream truck. The other kids cheered him on, their excitement palpable in the air.

And so, with a mischievous grin plastered across his face, Timmy took the wheel and revved the engine, his tiny feet barely reaching the pedals. The ice cream truck lurched forward, much to the shock and horror of the driver, who stood frozen in place, his mouth agape like a fish out of water.

What followed was a scene straight out of a slapstick comedy. The ice cream truck, now under the command of pint-sized pirates, embarked on a slow-speed chase through the streets of Sunnyvale, with the bewildered driver in hot pursuit, his shouts of protest falling on deaf ears.

Round and round they went, like a merry-go-round gone mad, the kids in the truck laughing uproariously as they swerved and dodged obstacles with all the finesse of seasoned race car drivers. Meanwhile, the driver, red-faced and sweating profusely, struggled to keep up, his attempts to catch the runaway truck resembling a wacky cartoon chase scene.

Eventually, after what felt like an eternity of laughter and chaos, the ice cream truck came to a halt, its pint-sized hijackers collapsing into fits of giggles as the driver finally caught up, panting and wheezing like a tired old steam engine.

And so, amidst the chaos and laughter, the Great Ice Cream Caper of 1956 came to an end, leaving the town of Sunnyvale with a tale to tell for generations to come. And as for the ice cream truck driver? Well, let's just say he never left his truck unattended again.

The Quirky Quack-Up: The Case of the Dancing Duck

In the sleepy town of Featherfield, nestled amidst rolling hills and babbling brooks, there lived a farmer named Old MacDonald. Now, Old MacDonald wasn't your ordinary farmer; he had a peculiar duck named Daffy, whose antics would have put even the most seasoned comedians to shame.

One fine morning in the spring of 1952, as the sun peeked over the horizon like a curious cat, Old MacDonald ventured out to tend to his farm chores. Little did he know, he was about to stumble upon a mystery that would have the whole town quacking with laughter.

As Old MacDonald approached the duck pond, he noticed something peculiar: Daffy, his feathered friend, was waddling around in circles, flapping his wings and bobbing his head in what appeared to be a peculiar dance.

Old MacDonald rubbed his eyes in disbelief, wondering if the early morning dew had played tricks on his vision. But no, there was no mistaking it—Daffy the duck was dancing like there was no tomorrow, his webbed feet tapping out a rhythm that would have made Fred Astaire proud.

Word of the dancing duck spread like wildfire through the town of Featherfield, drawing curious onlookers from far and wide. Soon, a crowd had gathered by the duck pond, their eyes wide with wonder as they watched Daffy's impromptu dance performance unfold.

The local newspaper even sent out a reporter to cover the story, penning headlines that read, "Featherfield's Funkiest Fowl: The Duck Who Danced His Way into Hearts."

As the days passed, Daffy's dancing prowess only seemed to improve, with each routine more intricate and awe-inspiring than the last. He twirled, he shuffled, he even attempted the moonwalk (albeit with limited success), much to the delight of the adoring crowd.

Speculation ran rampant throughout the town as to the cause of Daffy's newfound talent. Some claimed it was the result of a diet rich in breadcrumbs and birdseed, while others swore it was simply a case of duck fever catching on.

But the truth, as it turned out, was far simpler (and sillier) than anyone could have imagined. One day, as Old MacDonald sat by the duck pond, strumming his banjo and humming a merry tune, he noticed something peculiar: every time he played a certain melody, Daffy would start to dance.

It seemed that Daffy had developed a fondness for music, and Old MacDonald's banjo playing was the key to unlocking his inner dancing duck. From that day forward, Old MacDonald became known as the Pied Piper of Poultry, his banjo serenades drawing crowds from far and wide to witness Daffy's dazzling dance routines.

And so, amidst laughter and applause, Featherfield embraced its quirky quack-up: The Case of the Dancing Duck, a tale that would go down in history as one of the town's most cherished and comical mysteries. And as for Daffy? Well, let's just say he danced his way into the hearts of everyone he met, proving that sometimes, the silliest mysteries are the ones worth celebrating the most.

The Chicken Who Laid Square Eggs

In the quaint village of Eggsville, where the sun rose with a golden yawn and the roosters crowed like enthusiastic alarm clocks, there lived a farmer named Farmer Brown. Now, Farmer Brown wasn't your average farmer; he had a hen named Henrietta who was as peculiar as a three-legged cow.

One sunny morning in the summer of 1953, as Farmer Brown went about his daily chores, he stumbled upon a sight that nearly made his eyes pop out of his head like popped corn kernels. There, nestled snugly in Henrietta's coop, were not the usual oval-shaped eggs, but perfectly square ones!

Farmer Brown blinked in disbelief, wondering if he had accidentally stumbled into the plot of a science fiction novel. But no, there was no mistaking it—the eggs were unmistakably square, with sharp corners and straight edges that defied all laws of poultry physics.

Word of Henrietta's square eggs spread like wildfire through the village of Eggsville, drawing curious onlookers from far and wide. Soon, the once-quiet farm was overrun with visitors, all clamoring to catch a glimpse of the chicken who had laid the most peculiar eggs in all the land.

The local newspaper even sent out a reporter to cover the story, penning headlines that read, "Eggsville's Edgiest Eggs: The Chicken Who Thinks Outside the Oval."

As speculation ran rampant throughout the village as to the cause of Henrietta's square eggs, Farmer Brown found himself at a loss for answers. Some claimed it was the result of a bizarre genetic mutation, while others insisted it was simply a case of chicken shenanigans gone awry.

But the truth, as it turned out, was far simpler (and sillier) than anyone could have imagined. One day, as Farmer Brown sat scratching his head and pondering the mystery of Henrietta's square eggs, he noticed something peculiar: every time Henrietta laid an egg, she would give a little squawk and then do a little dance—a dance that just so happened to involve marching in perfectly straight lines and turning at precise right angles.

It seemed that Henrietta had developed a fondness for geometry, and her penchant for precision was the key to her peculiar eggs. From that day forward, Farmer Brown became known as the Architect of Agriculture, his farm drawing crowds from far and wide to witness Henrietta's egg-laying acrobatics.

And so, amidst laughter and applause, Eggsville embraced its clucking conundrum: The Chicken Who Laid Square Eggs, a tale that would go down in history as one of the village's most cherished and comical mysteries. And as for Henrietta? Well, let's just say she strutted around the farmyard with her head held high, proving that sometimes, the most unexpected surprises come in the most unexpected shapes.

The Great TP Tango: A Tale of Toilet Paper Panic

In the bustling town of Wipeaway, where the streets were lined with fluffy clouds and the laughter of children echoed like giggling geese, there occurred a calamity of colossal proportions: The Great Toilet Paper Shortage Panic of 1957.

It all began innocently enough, on a crisp autumn morning, when Mrs. Jenkins, the town gossip extraordinaire, let slip a whispered rumor that sent shockwaves through the community faster than a speeding roll of Charmin. "They say there's a shortage of toilet paper!" she exclaimed, her voice trembling with a mixture of horror and fascination.

At first, the townsfolk dismissed Mrs. Jenkins' words as nothing more than idle gossip, like the ramblings of a chicken with its feathers ruffled. But soon, the rumor took on a life of its own, spreading like wildfire through the town faster than a toddler with a roll of tape.

Before long, the streets of Wipeaway were flooded with panicked shoppers, their arms laden with rolls of toilet paper like precious treasure, their eyes wide with fear at the thought of a world without the soft embrace of two-ply goodness.

Supermarkets resembled battlegrounds, with shoppers engaged in fierce skirmishes over the last remaining rolls, their cries of "Mine!" and "Hands off my Charmin!" echoing through the aisles like battle cries.

Meanwhile, back at home, families resorted to desperate measures to cope with the impending crisis. Some stockpiled rolls by the dozen, hoarding them away like squirrels with their precious nuts. Others turned to creative alternatives, fashioning makeshift toilet paper out of newspaper, leaves, and even the occasional sock (much to the dismay of their feet).

The local newspaper even ran headlines declaring, "Wipeaway in Turmoil: Toilet Paper Tumult Takes Town by Storm!"

But amidst the chaos and confusion, there were moments of levity and laughter that served as a reminder of the resilience of the human spirit. Neighbors banded together, sharing rolls of toilet paper like precious gold, and swapping stories of their most memorable bathroom escapades.

As quickly as it had begun, the Toilet Paper Shortage Panic of 1957 came to an end, leaving the town of Wipeaway with a tale to tell for generations to come. And though the shelves may have been empty and the streets may have been littered with discarded cardboard tubes, the spirit of Wipeaway remained unbroken, a testament to the power of laughter in the face of adversity.

And so, as the sun set over the town of Wipeaway, casting a warm glow over its streets and alleys, the townsfolk breathed a collective sigh of relief, grateful for the soft touch of two-ply bliss and the reminder that sometimes, a little laughter is the best medicine for a world gone mad over toilet paper.

Briefs in Bloom: The Great Underwear Hoax

In the sleepy suburb of Cottonville, where the clotheslines swayed in the breeze like rhythmic dancers and the scent of fabric softener hung heavy in the air, there occurred a scandal of epic proportions: The Great Underwear Hoax of 1954.

It all began innocently enough, on a sunny Saturday morning, when Mrs. Smith, the town's resident busybody, happened upon a sight that left her jaw hanging lower than a pair of boxer shorts on a clothesline. There, fluttering in the gentle breeze, were not the usual array of socks and shirts, but thousands upon thousands of brightly colored underwear—boxers, briefs, bloomers, and everything in between—strung up like a technicolor tapestry.

At first, Mrs. Smith assumed it was simply a case of laundry day gone wild, a momentary lapse in judgment on the part of Cottonville's laundry aficionados. But as she wandered through the streets, her eyes wide with disbelief, she realized that this was no ordinary laundry mishap—this was a full-blown underwear uprising.

Word of the spectacle spread like wildfire through the town, drawing curious onlookers from far and wide. Soon, the streets of Cottonville were abuzz with whispers and giggles as the townsfolk gathered to marvel at the spectacle unfolding before their eyes.

The local newspaper even ran headlines declaring, "Underwear Uproar Unfolds: Cottonville in Stitches Over Spectacular Sighting!"

But amidst the laughter and confusion, there were whispers of suspicion and speculation as to the cause of the underwear uprising. Some claimed it was the work of mischievous teenagers, pulling off the prank of the century with a few rolls of duct tape and a whole lot of underwear. Others pointed fingers at extraterrestrial forces, suggesting that aliens with a penchant for unmentionables had descended upon Cottonville in search of the perfect pair of briefs.

But the truth, as it turned out, was far simpler (and sillier) than anyone could have imagined. One day, as the townsfolk gathered to admire the colorful spectacle before them, they noticed something peculiar: every pair of underwear bore a handwritten note attached with a safety pin, each one declaring in bold, block letters, "FREE UNDERWEAR FOR ALL!"

It seemed that the mysterious benefactor behind the underwear uprising had simply wanted to spread a little joy and laughter in a world that could always use a bit more of both. And spread joy it did, as the townsfolk danced and laughed amidst the sea of fluttering underwear, their hearts light and their spirits high.

And so, as the sun dipped below the horizon, casting a warm glow over Cottonville's streets and alleys, the townsfolk bid farewell to the Great Underwear Hoax of 1954, grateful for the laughter it had brought and the reminder that sometimes, the silliest pranks are the ones worth celebrating the most.

Gone in a Flash: The Mystery of the Vanishing Car

In the bustling town of Wheelsville, where the streets buzzed with the hum of engines and the scent of gasoline hung heavy in the air, there occurred a mystery of mammoth proportions: The Mystery of the Vanishing Car.

It all began on a foggy Friday evening, as Mr. Johnson, a local car enthusiast, parked his prized possession—a sleek, cherry-red convertible named Ruby—outside the local diner. Little did he know, he was about to become embroiled in a mystery that would have the whole town scratching their heads in confusion.

As Mr. Johnson emerged from the diner, his belly full of burgers and his heart light with contentment, he couldn't believe his eyes. There, in the spot where he had parked Ruby mere moments before, was nothing but an empty space—a void of asphalt where his beloved car should have been.

Mr. Johnson blinked in disbelief, wondering if he had accidentally stumbled onto the set of a magician's stage show. But no, there was no mistaking it—Ruby was gone, vanished into thin air like a puff of smoke on a windy day.

Word of the spectacle spread like wildfire through the town, drawing curious onlookers from far and wide. Soon, the streets of Wheelsville were abuzz with whispers and rumors as the townsfolk gathered to marvel at the mysterious disappearance.

The local newspaper even ran headlines declaring, "Wheels Gone Wild: Wheelsville in a Spin Over Vanishing Vehicle!"

But amidst the confusion and chaos, there were moments of levity and laughter as the townsfolk pondered the absurdity of the situation. Some speculated that Ruby had been abducted by aliens in search of the perfect getaway vehicle, while others suggested that she had simply grown tired of life in the fast lane and taken off on a solo adventure.

But the truth, as it turned out, was far simpler (and sillier) than anyone could have imagined. One day, as the townsfolk gathered to commiserate over the disappearance of Ruby, they noticed something peculiar: parked in the spot where Ruby had once stood was a shiny new scooter, its handlebars gleaming in the sunlight and a note attached to its seat that read, "Sorry for the mix-up—hope this makes up for it! Love, Ruby."

It seemed that Ruby had simply decided to trade in her four wheels for two, embarking on a new adventure in style. And while Mr. Johnson may have been initially perplexed by the disappearance of his beloved car, he couldn't help but chuckle at the absurdity of it all.

And so, as the sun set over the town of Wheelsville, casting a warm glow over its streets and alleys, the townsfolk bid farewell to the Mystery of the Vanishing Car, grateful for the laughter it had brought and the reminder that sometimes, the silliest mysteries are the ones worth celebrating the most.

The Canine Comedian: The Tale of the Talking Dog

In the quaint suburb of Barksville, where the trees whispered secrets to the wind and the squirrels danced like acrobats in the treetops, there lived a family named the Johnsons. Now, the Johnsons were your typical suburban family—two kids, a picket fence, and a dog named Max who was as ordinary as they come, or so they thought.

One fine day in the summer of 1953, as Mr. Johnson was puttering around the garden and Mrs. Johnson was hanging laundry on the line, they were interrupted by an unexpected sight: Max, their lovable mutt, was sitting on the front porch, chatting away like a seasoned conversationalist.

"Good day, Mr. and Mrs. Johnson!" Max exclaimed, his tail wagging furiously as he grinned up at them with a toothy grin.

Mr. and Mrs. Johnson blinked in disbelief, wondering if the heat had finally gotten to them or if they had accidentally stumbled into the plot of a children's storybook. But no, there was no mistaking it—Max was talking, and he had quite a lot to say.

Word of the spectacle spread like wildfire through the neighborhood, drawing curious onlookers from far and wide. Soon, the streets of Barksville were abuzz with whispers and giggles as the townsfolk gathered to marvel at the sight of Max, the talking dog.

The local newspaper even ran headlines declaring, "Barking Up the Right Tree: Barksville's Canine Comedian Leaves Town in Stitches!"

But amidst the laughter and confusion, there were whispers of suspicion and speculation as to the cause of Max's newfound talent. Some claimed it was the result of a bizarre scientific experiment gone awry, while others insisted it was simply a case of a dog with a knack for comedy.

But the truth, as it turned out, was far simpler (and sillier) than anyone could have imagined. One day, as the townsfolk gathered to hear Max's latest jokes and anecdotes, they noticed something peculiar: every time Max opened his mouth to speak, he would produce a sound that bore a striking resemblance to a kazoo—a high-pitched, squeaky noise that set off fits of laughter wherever he went.

It seemed that Max had discovered his inner comedian, and his talent for talking was simply a case of a dog with a flair for the dramatic. From that day forward, Barksville became known as the home of the talking dog, a town where laughter echoed through the streets and Max's kazoo-like banter brought joy to all who heard it.

And so, as the sun set over the town of Barksville, casting a warm glow over its streets and alleys, the townsfolk bid farewell to the Tale of the Talking Dog, grateful for the laughter it had brought and the reminder that sometimes, the silliest stories are the ones worth telling the most.

The Case of the Missing Pie: A Sweet Mystery Unraveled

In the cozy town of Sweetville, where the air was always filled with the aroma of freshly baked pies and the sound of laughter floated through the streets like butterflies on a breeze, there lived a mischievous character known far and wide as the Notorious Pie Thief.

Now, the Notorious Pie Thief wasn't your ordinary troublemaker; he had a reputation for swiping pies faster than a squirrel snatching acorns. No pie was safe from his sticky fingers, and no baker could outwit his insatiable appetite for sweet treats.

One sunny afternoon in the summer of 1955, as Mrs. Smith, the town's most renowned pie baker, was busy tending to her oven, she heard a rustling sound coming from her kitchen window. Peeking through the curtains, she was greeted by a sight that left her gasping in disbelief: the Notorious Pie Thief, his face smeared with cherry filling and a mischievous twinkle in his eye, making off with her prized apple pie.

Mrs. Smith blinked in astonishment, wondering if she had accidentally stumbled upon the plot of a slapstick comedy. But no, there was no mistaking it—the Notorious Pie Thief had struck again, leaving behind a trail of crumbs and chaos in his wake.

Word of the spectacle spread like wildfire through the town, drawing curious onlookers from far and wide. Soon, the streets of Sweetville were abuzz with whispers and giggles as the townsfolk gathered to marvel at the audacity of the Notorious Pie Thief.

The local newspaper even ran headlines declaring, "Sweetville's Sweetest Swindle: Notorious Pie Thief Strikes Again!"

But amidst the laughter and confusion, there were whispers of suspicion and speculation as to the identity of the Pie Thief. Some claimed it was a band of mischievous raccoons, while others insisted it was simply a case of pie-induced madness.

But the truth, as it turned out, was far simpler (and sillier) than anyone could have imagined. One day, as the townsfolk gathered to commiserate over the disappearance of Mrs. Smith's apple pie, they noticed something peculiar: every time the Pie Thief struck, there was a trail of flour leading straight to the culprit's hideout—a treehouse nestled high in the branches of the tallest oak tree in Sweetville.

It seemed that the Notorious Pie Thief was none other than Little Timmy, the town's most notorious troublemaker, whose love for pies knew no bounds. From that day forward, Sweetville became known as the home of the Pie Thief, a town where laughter and mischief danced hand in hand and every pie had to be guarded like treasure.

And so, as the sun set over the town of Sweetville, casting a warm glow over its streets and alleys, the townsfolk bid farewell to the Case of the Missing Pie, grateful for the laughter it had brought and the reminder that sometimes, the sweetest mysteries are the ones worth solving the most.

The Alien Antics: A Close Encounter of the Mischief Kind

In the sleepy town of Starlight Hills, where the nights were as dark as a cow's belly and the stars twinkled like mischievous fireflies, there occurred a curious event that left the townsfolk scratching their heads and reaching for their tin foil hats: The UFO Sighting Hoax of 1958.

It all began one moonlit night, as the Johnson family was enjoying a backyard barbecue beneath the twinkling sky. Suddenly, young Billy Johnson pointed up at the heavens and shouted, "Look! A UFO!"

His parents and neighbors gazed skyward in astonishment, their eyes wide with wonder as they spotted a strange, glowing object hovering in the distance like a giant disco ball.

Word of the sighting spread like wildfire through the town, drawing curious onlookers from far and wide. Soon, the streets of Starlight Hills were abuzz with whispers and speculation as the townsfolk gathered to marvel at the supposed extraterrestrial visitation.

The local newspaper even ran headlines declaring, "Out of This World: Starlight Hills in a Spin Over UFO Sighting!"

But amidst the excitement and confusion, there were whispers of suspicion and skepticism as to the authenticity of the UFO sighting. Some claimed it was simply a case of swamp gas or a weather balloon mistaken for an alien spacecraft, while others insisted it was the real deal—a visitation from beings beyond the stars.

But the truth, as it turned out, was far simpler (and sillier) than anyone could have imagined. One day, as the townsfolk gathered to discuss the mysterious sighting, they noticed something peculiar: hidden behind a nearby hill was a group of mischievous teenagers, giggling and whispering amongst themselves.

It seemed that the UFO sighting was nothing more than a prank orchestrated by the teens, who had crafted a makeshift flying saucer out of tin foil and string to fool the unsuspecting townsfolk. And fool them they did, as the sight of their makeshift UFO sent the town of Starlight Hills into a frenzy of excitement and speculation.

From that day forward, Starlight Hills became known as the town that had a close encounter of the mischief kind, a place where laughter and silliness were just as likely to be found in the night sky as stars and planets.

And so, as the sun set over the town of Starlight Hills, casting a warm glow over its streets and alleys, the townsfolk bid farewell to the UFO Sighting Hoax, grateful for the laughter it had brought and the reminder that sometimes, the most extraordinary events can have the most ordinary explanations.

Trunk Trouble: The Tale of the Escaped Circus Elephant

In the bustling town of Big Topville, where the air was filled with the scent of popcorn and the sound of laughter echoed like a symphony, there occurred a spectacle of mammoth proportions: The Escaped Circus Elephant.

It all began one sunny afternoon, as the Big Top Circus was setting up for its grand performance. Amidst the flurry of activity, a mischievous elephant named Ellie had plans of her own. With a mischievous twinkle in her eye and a swish of her mighty trunk, Ellie broke free from her enclosure and embarked on an adventure that would have the whole town talking for years to come.

As Ellie rumbled through the streets of Big Topville, her fellow circus performers raced to catch up, their cries of "Stop, Ellie, stop!" drowned out by the sounds of her thunderous footsteps and the delighted laughter of the townsfolk.

Word of the spectacle spread like wildfire through the town, drawing curious onlookers from far and wide. Soon, the streets of Big Topville were abuzz with whispers and giggles as the townsfolk gathered to marvel at the sight of Ellie, the runaway circus elephant.

The local newspaper even ran headlines declaring, "Big Top Chaos: Elephant Escapade Leaves Town in Stitches!"

But amidst the chaos and confusion, there were moments of levity and laughter as the townsfolk watched Ellie's antics unfold. Some claimed she was on a mission to find the world's largest peanut, while others insisted she was simply tired of the same old circus routine and yearned for a taste of freedom.

But the truth, as it turned out, was far simpler (and sillier) than anyone could have imagined. One day, as the townsfolk gathered to witness Ellie's grand adventure, they noticed something peculiar: perched atop Ellie's mighty back was a tiny mouse, steering her through the streets with all the finesse of a seasoned circus performer.

It seemed that Ellie's escapade was nothing more than a game of cat and mouse, with the mischievous mouse leading her on a merry chase through the streets of Big Topville. And chase her they did, as the sight of Ellie and her tiny accomplice sent the town into fits of laughter and applause.

From that day forward, Big Topville became known as the town that had a close encounter with the pachyderm kind, a place where laughter and silliness were just as likely to be found in the streets as under the big top.

And so, as the sun set over the town of Big Topville, casting a warm glow over its streets and alleys, the townsfolk bid farewell to Ellie's grand escapade, grateful for the laughter it had brought and the reminder that sometimes, the most extraordinary adventures can have the most ordinary explanations.

The Mischievous Monkey Mischief: A Whimsical Tale of an Escaped Primate

Once upon a time, in the bustling town of Riverside, where trees whispered secrets and laughter echoed through the streets like a symphony of silliness, there occurred an event that would go down in history as The Case of the Escaped Monkey.

It all started with a curious little monkey named Benny, who lived at the local zoo. Benny was a mischievous creature with a penchant for adventure and one sunny afternoon, he decided to embark on a daring escapade.

The local news ran headlines declaring, "Riverside's Rambunctious Rascal: The Case of the Escaped Monkey Leaves Town in a Tizzy of Treetop Tomfoolery!"

But amidst the chaos and confusion, there were moments of sheer hilarity as Benny frolicked through the town, swinging from lampposts and teasing passersby with his playful antics. Some gasped in surprise, while others chuckled at the sight of the cheeky monkey in a comical display of primate pandemonium.

But the true heroes of the day were a group of animal enthusiasts known as the Zookeepers' Zealots, who had unwittingly become the champions of Riverside's monkey mayhem with their ingenious tactics and quick thinking. With each banana bait and each coaxing call, they brought joy and laughter to all who joined in the monkey mischief.

From that day forward, Riverside became known as the town that had a close encounter with the monkey kind, a place where even the most unexpected of events could bring people together in laughter and camaraderie.

And so, as the residents of Riverside bid farewell to The Case of the Escaped Monkey and continued to reminisce about Benny's misadventures with a smile on their faces and a twinkle in their eyes, they did so knowing that they had been part of a truly hilarious and unforgettable primate escapade.

The Out-of-This-World Prank: A Whimsical Tale of the Great "Flying Saucer" Hoax

Once upon a time, in the quiet town of Pineview, where cows grazed lazily and birds chirped merrily, there occurred an event that would go down in history as The Great "Flying Saucer" Hoax.

It all started on a dark and stormy night when the mischievous Smith brothers, Tom and Tim, concocted a harebrained scheme to prank their neighbors. Armed with aluminum foil, string lights, and a healthy dose of imagination, they set out to create a spectacle that would leave the town buzzing.

The local news ran headlines declaring, "Pineview's Preposterous Prank: The Great 'Flying Saucer' Hoax Leaves Town in a Tizzy of Extraterrestrial Excitement!"

But amidst the chaos and confusion, there were moments of sheer hilarity as the townsfolk gazed up at the sky, wide-eyed and bewildered by the sight of the "flying saucer" hovering above. Some gasped in astonishment, while others scratched their heads in disbelief at the otherworldly apparition in a comical display of extraterrestrial enthusiasm.

But the true heroes of the day were none other than the Smith brothers themselves, who had unwittingly become the champions of Pineview's prankster pantheon with their audacious antics and creative flair. With each flicker of the lights and each gasp of amazement, they brought joy and laughter to all who joined in the flying saucer frenzy.

From that day forward, Pineview became known as the town that had a close encounter of the hoax kind, a place where even the most outlandish of pranks could bring people together in laughter and camaraderie.

And so, as the residents of Pineview bid farewell to The Great "Flying Saucer" Hoax and continued to regale each other with tales of the Smith brothers' shenanigans, they did so with a smile on their faces and a twinkle in their eyes, knowing that they had been part of a truly hilarious and unforgettable extraterrestrial escapade.

The Clucking Conundrum: A Feathered Tale of the Mystery of the Dancing Chicken

Once upon a time, in the bustling farmyard of Sunnyvale, where roosters crowed and pigs oinked, there occurred an event that would go down in history as The Mystery of the Dancing Chicken.

It all started one bright and sunny morning when Farmer Joe discovered something peculiar in his chicken coop. There, amidst the clucking hens and pecking chicks, was Henrietta, his prize-winning chicken, doing a jig that would put even the most seasoned dancers to shame.

The local news ran headlines declaring, "Sunnyvale's Startling Surprise: The Mystery of the Dancing Chicken Leaves Town in a Tizzy of Twirls and Twists!"

But amidst the confusion and bewilderment, there were moments of sheer hilarity as the townsfolk gathered around to witness Henrietta's impromptu dance performance. Some clapped their hands in delight, while others scratched their heads in wonder at the sight of the dancing chicken in a comical display of barnyard befuddlement.

But the true hero of the day was none other than Henrietta herself, who had unwittingly become the star of Sunnyvale's feathered flock with her fancy footwork and undeniable charm. With each graceful step and each elegant twirl, she brought joy and laughter to all who watched her dance.

From that day forward, Sunnyvale became known as the town that had a close encounter with the clucking kind, a place where even the most unlikely of creatures could bust a move and bring people together in laughter and camaraderie.

And so, as the residents of Sunnyvale bid farewell to The Mystery of the Dancing Chicken and continued to marvel at Henrietta's antics with a smile on their faces and a chuckle in their hearts, they did so knowing that they had been part of a truly hilarious and unforgettable barnyard adventure.

The Tail of the Three-Legged Cat: A Whimsical Tale of Feline Frolics

Once upon a time, in the cozy neighborhood of Maplewood, where trees whispered secrets and squirrels chattered like gossiping neighbors, there lived a cat named Tripod. Tripod was no ordinary cat – he was a three-legged wonder, known far and wide for his hilarious hijinks.

It all started when Tripod, with his playful spirit and boundless energy, would chase after mice with a vigor that belied his missing limb. The local news ran headlines declaring, "Maplewood's Marvelous Mischief: The Hilarious Hijinks of the Three-Legged Cat Leaves Town in Stitches!"

But amidst the laughter and amusement, there were moments of sheer hilarity as Tripod navigated his world with a unique blend of determination and clumsiness. Some marveled at his acrobatic feats, while others chuckled at his occasional tumbles in a comical display of feline folly.

But the true hero of the day was none other than Tripod himself, who had unwittingly become the star of Maplewood's pet parade with his antics and charm. With each playful pounce and each daring leap, he brought joy and laughter to all who watched him.

From that day forward, Maplewood became known as the town that had a close encounter of the whiskered kind, a place where even a three-legged cat could bring people together in laughter and camaraderie.

And so, as the residents of Maplewood bid farewell to The Hilarious Hijinks of the Three-Legged Cat and continued to regale each other with tales of Tripod's adventures, they did so with a smile on their faces and a purr in their hearts, knowing that they had been part of a truly hilarious and unforgettable feline frolic.

The Invisible Dog Debacle: A Hilarious Tale of Imaginary Antics

Once upon a time, in the lively neighborhood of Oakwood, where trees whispered secrets and children laughed like music in the air, there occurred an event that would go down in history as The Absurdity of the "Invisible Dog" Prank.

It all started when young Tommy, armed with nothing but a leash and a mischievous grin, decided to play a prank on his unsuspecting neighbors. Pretending to walk an invisible dog named Fido, Tommy strutted down the sidewalk with all the confidence of a seasoned pet owner.

The local news ran headlines declaring, "Oakwood's Outrageous Omission: The Absurdity of the 'Invisible Dog' Prank Leaves Town in a Tizzy of Tail-Wagging Tales!"

But amidst the confusion and laughter, there were moments of sheer hilarity as passersby watched in amazement at Tommy's antics. Some gasped in astonishment, while others doubled over in laughter at the sight of the imaginary pooch in a comical display of canine confusion.

But the true hero of the day was none other than Tommy himself, who had unwittingly become the star of Oakwood's invisible menagerie with his imaginative prank. With each tug of the leash and each playful bark, he brought joy and laughter to all who witnessed his invisible dog walk.

From that day forward, Oakwood became known as the neighborhood that had a close encounter of the transparent kind, a place where even the most absurd of pranks could bring people together in laughter and camaraderie.

And so, as the residents of Oakwood bid farewell to The Absurdity of the "Invisible Dog" Prank and continued to reminisce about Tommy's imaginary antics with a smile on their faces and a chuckle in their hearts, they did so knowing that they had been part of a truly hilarious and unforgettable neighborhood escapade.

The Pie-Eating Fiasco: A Legendary Tale of Culinary Chaos

Once upon a time, in the quaint town of Cherryville, where cherry trees bloomed and pies filled the air with their tantalizing aroma, there occurred an event that would go down in history as The Legendary Pie-Eating Contest Mishap.

It all started on a sunny Saturday afternoon when the townsfolk gathered in the town square for the annual pie-eating contest. The local news ran headlines declaring, "Cherryville's Culinary Catastrophe: The Legendary Pie-Eating Contest Mishap Leaves Town in a Sweet Mess!"

But amidst the excitement and anticipation, there were moments of sheer hilarity as contestants dove face-first into their pies with reckless abandon. Some slurped and slopped, while others chomped and chewed in a comical display of culinary chaos.

But the true hero of the day was none other than Billy, a young boy with an insatiable appetite and a penchant for mischief. With each bite and each gulp, he devoured his way through pie after pie, leaving a trail of whipped cream and fruit filling in his wake.

As the contest drew to a close and the judges tallied the scores, it became apparent that Billy had consumed far more than his fair share of pies. He had eaten every single pie in sight, much to the shock and amusement of the crowd.

From that day forward, Cherryville became known as the town that had a close encounter of the pastry kind, a place where even the most absurd of mishaps could bring people together in laughter and camaraderie.

And so, as the residents of Cherryville bid farewell to The Legendary Pie-Eating Contest Mishap and continued to reminisce about Billy's epic feat with a smile on their faces and a rumble in their stomachs, they did so knowing that they had been part of a truly hilarious and unforgettable culinary caper.

The Quacking Canine Companion: A Tail-Wagging Tale of Unlikely Friendship

In the serene countryside of Willow Grove, where grass swayed and ponds shimmered under the sun, an unlikely friendship blossomed between a dog named Max and a duck named Daisy. Their story, filled with whimsy and wonder, would warm the hearts of all who heard it.

Max, a friendly golden retriever with a wagging tail and a playful spirit, first encountered Daisy, a curious duckling, by the edge of the pond one sunny afternoon. The local news ran headlines declaring, "Willow Grove's Wonderful Waterfowl Wonders: The Unlikely Friendship Between a Dog and a Duck Leaves Town in High Spirits!"

But amidst the laughter and joy, there were moments of sheer hilarity as Max and Daisy embarked on their adventures together. Some marveled at their odd couple antics, while others chuckled at their playful pursuits in a comical display of interspecies camaraderie.

But the true magic of their friendship lay in the bond they shared—a bond that transcended differences and brought joy to all who witnessed it. With each wag of Max's tail and each quack of Daisy's beak, they reminded everyone that friendship knows no bounds.

From that day forward, Willow Grove became known as the town that had a close encounter with the furry and feathery kind, a place where even the most unlikely of friendships could bring people together in laughter and camaraderie.

And so, as the residents of Willow Grove bid farewell to The Unlikely Friendship Between a Dog and a Duck and continued to cherish the memories of Max and Daisy's adventures, they did so with a smile on their faces and a quack in their hearts, knowing that they had been part of a truly heartwarming and unforgettable tale.

The Sock Puppet Spectacle: An Unforgettable Tale of Whimsy and Wonder

Once upon a time, in the cozy town of Cottonwood, where laughter filled the air and creativity knew no bounds, there stood an old, forgotten sock drawer. Little did the townsfolk know, this drawer held the key to a magical world known as The Infamous "Sock Puppet" Theater.

It all began when a group of friends stumbled upon the dusty drawer one rainy afternoon. The local news ran headlines declaring, "Cottonwood's Comical Conundrum: The Infamous 'Sock Puppet' Theater Leaves Town in Stitches!"

But amidst the giggles and guffaws, there were moments of pure enchantment as the sock puppets came to life on the makeshift stage. Some marveled at the intricate performances, while others chuckled at the hilarious antics in a comical display of sock puppetry.

But the true magic of the theater lay in the boundless imagination of its creators—a group of friends who brought joy to all who watched their whimsical productions. With each flutter of fabric and each flick of felt, they transported their audience to a world of wonder and laughter.

From that day forward, Cottonwood became known as the town that had a close encounter of the sock puppet kind, a place where even the most ordinary of objects could become extraordinary in the hands of creative minds.

And so, as the residents of Cottonwood bid farewell to The Infamous "Sock Puppet" Theater and continued to cherish the memories of their whimsical performances, they did so with a smile on their faces and a sock puppet on their hands, knowing that they had been part of a truly unforgettable tale of whimsy and wonder.

The Great Toilet Paper Caper: A Tale of Comical Chaos

In the bustling city of Milltown, where streets buzzed with activity and laughter echoed through the air, an absurd panic erupted one fateful day—the Great Toilet Paper Shortage. What began as a simple rumor quickly spiraled into a comical frenzy that left the town in stitches.

It all started when one resident claimed to have heard whispers of a looming toilet paper shortage. The local news ran headlines declaring, "Milltown's Outrageous Outcry: The Great Toilet Paper Shortage Leaves Town in a Tizzy!"

But amidst the chaos and confusion, there were moments of sheer hilarity as residents scrambled to stockpile toilet paper like it was gold. Some hoarded rolls by the dozen, while others fashioned makeshift masks and costumes out of the coveted paper in a comical display of panic-induced creativity.

But the true hero of the day was none other than Old Mrs. Jenkins, the local wise woman, who had seen her fair share of absurdities in her time. With a twinkle in her eye and a hearty chuckle, she reminded everyone that toilet paper shortages were nothing new and that laughter was the best remedy for panic.

From that day forward, Milltown became known as the town that had a close encounter of the paper kind, a place where even the most ridiculous of panics could bring people together in laughter and camaraderie.

And so, as the residents of Milltown bid farewell to The Great Toilet Paper Shortage and continued to chuckle at the absurdity of it all, they did so with a smile on their faces and a roll of toilet paper in hand, knowing that they had been part of a truly unforgettable tale of comical chaos.

The Hilarious Hijinks of the Amateur Talent Show

In the small town of Sunnydale, where community spirit thrived and laughter filled the air, an amateur talent show was organized to showcase the hidden talents of its residents. Little did they know, the show would become an uproarious comedy of errors that would leave the audience in stitches.

It all began with the enthusiastic participants who eagerly signed up to showcase their talents. The local news ran headlines declaring, "Sunnydale's Side-Splitting Spectacle: The Comedy of Errors at the Amateur Talent Show Leaves Town in Fits of Laughter!"

But amidst the excitement and anticipation, there were moments of sheer hilarity as the performances took unexpected twists and turns. Some singers hit hilariously off-key notes, while others attempted daring dance moves with less-than-graceful results. One participant even attempted to juggle but ended up dropping all the balls in a comical display of mishaps.

But the true stars of the show were the emcees, a pair of bumbling brothers who couldn't seem to get anything right. With each botched introduction and missed cue, they inadvertently stole the spotlight and had the audience roaring with laughter.

From that day forward, Sunnydale became known as the town that had a close encounter of the comedic kind, a place where even the most earnest of endeavors could turn into a sidesplitting spectacle.

And so, as the residents of Sunnydale bid farewell to The Comedy of Errors at the Amateur Talent Show and continued to chuckle at the memories, they did so with a smile on their faces and a newfound appreciation for the joy of la

Let's go Back

To the 60's

The Bikini Bust: A Tale of the Great Swimsuit Ban

In the sunny seaside town of Sunburn Bay, where the waves kissed the shore and the seagulls sang songs of salty breezes, there occurred a tidal wave of controversy known far and wide as the Great Swimsuit Ban of 1964.

It all began one scorching summer day, as the town council convened for their monthly meeting. Amidst the sweltering heat and the buzz of cicadas, Mayor Thompson stood up and cleared his throat, his face flushed with determination.

"Ladies and gentlemen," he declared, his voice booming like a foghorn, "I propose a ban on swimsuits of a certain... revealing nature."

The townsfolk gasped in astonishment, their mouths agape like fish out of water. A ban on swimsuits? In Sunburn Bay? It was unheard of!

Word of the proposal spread like wildfire through the town, drawing curious onlookers from far and wide. Soon, the streets of Sunburn Bay were abuzz with whispers and giggles as the townsfolk debated the merits of the mayor's plan.

The local newspaper even ran headlines declaring, "Sunny Skies, Shady Swimsuits: Sunburn Bay in a Flurry Over Ban Proposal!"

But amidst the uproar and confusion, there were moments of levity and laughter as the townsfolk imagined a world without its beloved bikinis and trunks. Some claimed they would fashion swimsuits out of seaweed and seashells, while others joked about skinny dipping under the cover of darkness.

But the truth, as it turned out, was far simpler (and sillier) than anyone could have imagined. One day, as the townsfolk gathered to protest the proposed ban, they noticed something peculiar: perched atop the mayor's head was a seagull, squawking and flapping its wings with all the fervor of a town crier.

It seemed that the seagull had taken a liking to the mayor's straw hat and had decided to make it his perch for the day. And perch he did, as the sight of the mayor and his feathered friend sent the town into fits of laughter and applause.

From that day forward, Sunburn Bay became known as the town that had a brush with the bikini bust, a place where laughter and silliness were just as likely to be found on the beach as in the town square.

And so, as the sun set over the town of Sunburn Bay, casting a warm glow over its sandy shores and palm-lined streets, the townsfolk bid farewell to the Great Swimsuit Ban of 1964, grateful for the laughter it had brought and the reminder that sometimes, the silliest controversies are the ones worth laughing about the most.

Fab Four Fiasco: The Beatles' Pillow Fight Frenzy

In the swinging sixties of Liverpool, where the streets pulsed with the beat of rock and roll and the air was electric with the promise of revolution, there occurred a legendary event that would go down in history as the Fab Four Fiasco: The Beatles' Pillow Fight.

It all began one rainy afternoon in the spring of 1963, as John, Paul, George, and Ringo lounged in their hotel room, bored out of their minds and itching for a bit of excitement. With a mischievous gleam in their eyes and a twinkle of mischief in their hearts, they seized upon an idea that would send shockwaves through the world of music.

"Let's have a pillow fight!" exclaimed John, his Liverpudlian accent thick with excitement.

The other Beatles grinned and nodded in agreement, their enthusiasm contagious as they rummaged through the hotel's linen closet in search of the softest, fluffiest pillows they could find.

Word of the spectacle spread like wildfire through the hotel, drawing curious onlookers from far and wide. Soon, the corridors were filled with the sound of laughter and the sight of feathers flying as the Fab Four engaged in an epic battle of fluffy proportions.

The hotel staff watched in astonishment as John, Paul, George, and Ringo pelted each other with pillows, their laughter echoing through the halls like a symphony of silliness. Guests peeked out from their rooms, their eyes wide with wonder as they witnessed the spectacle unfolding before them.

The local newspaper even ran headlines declaring, "Beatlemania Strikes Again: Fab Four Fiasco Leaves Hotel in Shambles!"

But amidst the chaos and confusion, there were moments of pure joy and camaraderie as the Beatles reveled in their playful antics. They laughed until their sides ached and their cheeks hurt, their bonds as friends and bandmates stronger than ever before.

And as the sun set over the city of Liverpool, casting a warm glow over its streets and alleyways, the Beatles bid farewell to the Fab Four Fiasco, grateful for the laughter it had brought and the reminder that sometimes, even the biggest rock stars need to let loose and have a bit of fun.

Dolly Doppelgängers: The Hilarious Tale of the Look-Alike Contest

In the small town of Countryville, where the twang of guitars filled the air and cowboy boots were a staple of everyday attire, there occurred an event that would go down in history as the Dolly Parton Look-Alike Contest.

It all began one sunny Saturday afternoon at the local community center, where the townsfolk had gathered to celebrate their love for country music and all things Dolly. With her signature big hair, flashy outfits, and larger-than-life personality, Dolly Parton had long been a source of inspiration and admiration in Countryville.

As the contest got underway, the stage was soon filled with contestants vying for the title of Dolly's doppelgänger. There were men and women of all ages, each decked out in their finest Dolly-inspired attire, from sequined dresses to cowboy hats and everything in between.

The audience cheered and applauded as the contestants strutted their stuff, their attempts at channeling Dolly's iconic look ranging from spot-on to downright comical. Some sported wigs so big they threatened to topple over, while others flaunted outfits so bedazzled they could be seen from space.

The judges, a panel of local celebrities, and die-hard Dolly fans had their work cut out for them as they deliberated over who deserved the coveted title. They scribbled notes furiously, their faces contorted in concentration as they debated the finer points of Dolly's style and persona.

The tension in the air was palpable as the finalists were announced, their names echoing through the community center like a chorus of angels. With bated breath, the audience watched as each contestant took the stage once more, their eyes fixed on the prize and their hearts pounding with anticipation.

And then, finally, the moment of truth arrived: the winner of the Dolly Parton Look-Alike Contest was announced to thunderous applause and cheers. The lucky contestant, a sweet old grandma named Mildred, had captured Dolly's essence with her dazzling smile, sparkling eyes, and a wig so voluminous it could rival the Tennessee mountains.

As Mildred accepted her crown and sash with tears of joy streaming down her cheeks, she was greeted with hugs and kisses from her fellow contestants and adoring fans alike. As she took her place in the annals of Countryville history, she knew that she would forever be remembered as the queen of the Dolly Parton Look-Alike Contest, a title she wore with pride and a whole lot of country flair.

Mice in Space: The Hilarious Tale of NASA's Great Mouse Invasion

In the hallowed halls of NASA, where scientists worked tirelessly to unravel the mysteries of the cosmos and send humans soaring into the stars, there occurred an event that would go down in history as the Great Mouse Invasion.

It all began one ordinary day in the summer of 1969, as the scientists at NASA's headquarters in Houston, Texas, were hard at work preparing for the Apollo 11 moon landing. With the eyes of the world on them and the fate of the mission hanging in the balance, they were laser-focused on their tasks.

But little did they know, they were about to encounter a foe more fearsome than any they had faced before a horde of mischievous mice with a penchant for mischief and a hunger for adventure.

As the scientists toiled away in their labs and control rooms, they began to notice something peculiar: tiny squeaks and scurrying sounds echoing through the corridors, like whispers in the night. At first, they dismissed them as the harmless antics of a few stray rodents, but soon, the situation spiraled out of control.

Word of the mouse invasion spread like wildfire through NASA, drawing curious onlookers and concerned officials from far and wide. Soon, the halls were alive with the sound of traps snapping shut and scientists scrambling to catch the elusive critters before they could wreak havoc on the mission.

The local news ran headlines declaring, "Houston, We Have a Mouse Problem: NASA's Great Invasion Leaves Scientists Scratching Their Heads!"

But amidst the chaos and confusion, there were moments of levity and laughter as the scientists grappled with their unexpected visitors. Some joked about the mice stowing away on the Apollo spacecraft and embarking on a mission to the moon, while others marveled at their resilience and ingenuity.

But the truth, as it turned out, was far simpler (and sillier) than anyone could have imagined. One day, as the scientists were in the midst of a heated debate over the best way to rid NASA of its unwelcome guests, they noticed something peculiar: perched atop a pile of discarded papers was a tiny mouse, nibbling away at a crumb with all the gusto of a hungry astronaut.

It seemed that the mice had taken up residence in NASA's headquarters in search of adventure and a taste of the high life. And adventure they found, as they scurried through the corridors and explored every nook and cranny of the sprawling complex.

From that day forward, NASA became known as the space agency that had a close encounter with the furry kind, a place where even the tiniest creatures could leave a lasting impact on the course of history.

And so, as the scientists bid farewell to their uninvited guests and returned to their work with renewed determination, they knew that they would forever be remembered as the brave men and women who faced the Great Mouse Invasion of NASA with humor and grace.

The Sock Rebellion: A Hilarious Tale of the Great Sock Protest

Once upon a time, in the cozy town of Footsville, where the streets were paved with socks and the scent of laundry detergent filled the air, there occurred a revolution of epic proportions known far and wide as the Great Sock Protest.

It all began one dreary morning, as the residents of Footsville awoke to find their socks missing from their drawers and clotheslines. Panic ensued as they searched high and low for their missing footwear but to no avail. It seemed that the socks had vanished into thin air, leaving behind a town in turmoil.

But amidst the chaos, a brave group of socks refused to go quietly. Led by their fearless leader, a lone argyle sock named Socksy, they banded together to stage a protest against their disappearance.

The socks took to the streets, marching in single file with their mismatched pairs proudly on display. They carried signs that read "Sock Lives Matter" and "Give Us Our Freedom, Feet!" as they chanted slogans of defiance and solidarity.

Word of the protest spread like wildfire through Footsville, drawing curious onlookers and concerned authorities from far and wide. Soon, the streets were filled with spectators cheering on the socks as they made their voices heard.

The local news ran headlines declaring, "Sock It to 'Em: Footsville's Great Protest Leaves Town in Stitches!"

But amidst the laughter and confusion, there were moments of genuine emotion as the residents of Footsville realized the importance of their humble socks. They joined the protest in droves, marching alongside their socky comrades and demanding justice for all.

And justice they received, as it turned out that the socks had been spirited away by a mischievous group of laundry fairies in search of a good time. Upon learning of the socks' plight, the fairies returned them to Footsville with apologies and promised to never interfere with laundry day again.

From that day forward, Footsville became known as the town that stood up for its socks, a place where even the smallest garments could make a big difference.

And so, as the socks returned to their rightful place in drawers and clotheslines across Footsville, they knew that they had forever changed the course of history with their Great Sock Protest.

The Stinky Showdown: A Whiffy Tale of the Smelliest Football Game

In the town of Odorville, where the air was thick with the scent of sweat and the sound of cheers echoed through the streets, there occurred a football game that would go down in history as the Smelliest Football Game.

It all began one hot and humid afternoon, as the Odorville Stinkers and the Rotten Rivals faced off on the field for a showdown of epic proportions. The rivalry between the two teams was legendary, but little did they know, they were about to encounter a foe more formidable than any opponent they had faced before the dreaded stink bomb.

As the game got underway, the players raced across the field with reckless abandon, their noses wrinkled in disgust as they caught whiffs of the foul odor wafting through the air. It seemed that someone had unleashed a stink bomb onto the field, turning what should have been a friendly game of football into a battle of the senses.

The spectators gagged and choked on the noxious fumes as they watched the players soldier on, their eyes watering and their stomachs churning with every breath. The smell was so overpowering that even the referees had to hold their noses as they tried to keep the game under control.

The local news ran headlines declaring, "Foul Play: Odorville's Stinkiest Football Game Leaves Fans Holding Their Noses!"

But amidst the chaos and confusion, there were moments of sheer hilarity as the players struggled to navigate the field while holding their noses and gasping for fresh air. Some resorted to wearing clothespins on their noses, while others attempted to mask the smell with copious amounts of cologne.

But the truth, as it turned out, was far simpler (and sillier) than anyone could have imagined. One day, as the players and spectators alike were still reeling from the stench of the stink bomb, they noticed something peculiar: perched atop the goalposts was a flock of mischievous skunks, their tails raised high and their noses twitching with glee.

It seemed that the skunks had taken it upon themselves to spice up the game with their potent perfume, unaware of the chaos and confusion they were causing. And spice it up they did, as the sight of the skunks and their pungent aroma sent the town of Odorville into fits of laughter and applause.

From that day forward, Odorville became known as the town that had a close encounter with the smelly kind, a place where even the stinkiest situations could lead to laughter and camaraderie.

And so, as the players and spectators bid farewell to the Smelliest Football Game, they did so with smiles on their faces and memories of a game they would never forget.

Flamingo Fiasco: The Hilarious Tale of the Great Stolen Lawn Flamingo Caper

In the quiet suburb of Featherdale, where the lawns were manicured to perfection and the sound of birds chirping filled the air, there occurred an event that would go down in history as the Great Stolen Lawn Flamingo Caper.

It all began on a sunny afternoon, as Mrs. Jenkins stepped out onto her front porch to admire her prized collection of lawn flamingos. She had spent years curating the perfect flock, each flamingo painted in vibrant shades of pink and standing tall and proud on her perfectly manicured lawn.

But as Mrs. Jenkins surveyed her feathered friends, her heart skipped a beat. One of her beloved flamingos was missing! In its place was a lone feather, a cruel reminder of the feathered thief who had absconded with her prized possession.

Word of the theft spread like wildfire through Featherdale, drawing curious onlookers and concerned neighbors from far and wide. Soon, the streets were abuzz with whispers and speculation as the townsfolk tried to unravel the mystery of the missing flamingo.

The local news ran headlines declaring, "Featherdale's Fowl Play: Great Stolen Lawn Flamingo Caper Leaves Town in a Frenzy!"

But amidst the chaos and confusion, there were moments of levity and laughter as the townsfolk imagined the audacity of the flamingo thief.

Some speculated that it was a prank gone wrong, while others joked about the flamingo sprouting wings and flying away on its own.

But the truth, as it turned out, was far simpler (and sillier) than anyone could have imagined. One day, as Mrs. Jenkins was lamenting the loss of her beloved flamingo, she noticed something peculiar: perched atop her neighbor's roof was a mischievous cat, its fur tinged with streaks of pink paint and a guilty look in its eyes.

It seemed that the cat, in a fit of feline curiosity, had taken it upon itself to liberate the flamingo from Mrs. Jenkins' lawn and make it its own. And while Mrs. Jenkins may have been initially distraught by the loss of her flamingo, she couldn't help but chuckle at the absurdity of it all.

From that day forward, Featherdale became known as the town that had a close encounter with the feathered kind, a place where even the most mundane of objects could spark a mystery worthy of a detective novel.

And so, as Mrs. Jenkins bid farewell to her missing flamingo and welcomed it back into the flock with open arms (and a fresh coat of paint), she did so with a smile on her face and a newfound appreciation for the absurdity of life in Featherdale.

The Paw-litical Candidate: A Tail of the Poodle Who Ran for Mayor

In the quaint town of Pawsville, where the streets were lined with fire hydrants and the sound of barking filled the air, there occurred an event that would go down in history as the Paw-litical sensation of the century: The Poodle Who Ran for Mayor.

It all began one sunny afternoon, as the residents of Pawsville gathered in the town square for the annual pet parade. Among the parade participants was a fluffy white poodle named Fifi, whose impeccable grooming and charming demeanor had earned her the title of "Best in Show" for three years running.

But as Fifi pranced through the streets, her tail held high and her fur gleaming in the sunlight, she caught the eye of a group of local activists who were dissatisfied with the current state of affairs in Pawsville. With a bark of determination and a wag of her tail, Fifi declared her candidacy for mayor, much to the surprise and delight of the crowd.

Word of Fifi's candidacy spread like wildfire through Pawsville, drawing curious onlookers and eager supporters from far and wide. Soon, the town was buzzing with excitement as Fifi's campaign gained momentum, her face plastered on posters and her name on everyone's lips.

The local news ran headlines declaring, "Fur-tastic News: Pawsville's Paw-litical Scene Shaken Up by Poodle Mayor Candidacy!"

But amidst the excitement and anticipation, there were moments of levity and laughter as the townsfolk imagined what it would be like to have a poodle in the mayor's office. Some joked about Fifi instituting mandatory belly rub breaks, while others imagined her hosting extravagant "Yappy Hour" events in the town square.

But the truth, as it turned out, was far simpler (and sillier) than anyone could have imagined. One day, as the residents of Pawsville gathered to cast their votes in the mayoral election, they noticed something peculiar: perched atop the ballot box was a mischievous squirrel, its tail twitching with excitement as it nibbled on a peanut.

It seemed that the squirrel, in a bid to shake up the Paw-litical scene in Pawsville, had taken it upon itself to disrupt the election proceedings and throw a wrench into Fifi's campaign. While Fifi may not have emerged victorious in the end, she had succeeded in capturing the hearts and imaginations of the townsfolk, who would forever remember her as the poodle who dared to dream big.

From that day forward, Pawsville became known as the town that had a close encounter with the paw-litical kind, a place where even the smallest of creatures could make a big impact on the world around them.

And so, as Fifi bid farewell to her mayoral aspirations and returned to her life of luxury and leisure, she did so with a wag of her tail and a twinkle in her eye, knowing that she had left an indelible mark on the town of Pawsville and inspired a new generation of paw-litical activists to follow in her paw-steps.

The Elevator Escapade: A Hilarious Tale of the Great Stuck Elevator Incident

In the bustling city of Metropolis, where skyscrapers stretched towards the clouds and the streets teemed with people rushing to and fro, there occurred an event that would go down in history as the Great Stuck Elevator Incident.

It all began one ordinary morning, as a diverse group of Metropolis residents boarded the elevator of the city's tallest building, each with their destination in mind. Little did they know, they were about to embark on an unexpected journey that would test their patience, resilience, and sense of humor.

As the elevator began its ascent, the occupants chatted and joked amongst themselves, unaware of the impending calamity that awaited them. But then, with a sudden jolt and a groan of protest, the elevator came to a grinding halt, leaving its passengers stranded between floors.

Panic ensued as the occupants pressed frantically on the buttons and banged on the doors in a desperate bid for freedom. But try as they might, the elevator remained stubbornly stuck, its mechanical innards refusing to budge.

Word of the incident spread like wildfire through the building, drawing curious onlookers and concerned officials from far and wide. Soon, the lobby was filled with spectators peering up at the malfunctioning elevator with a mixture of amusement and sympathy.

The local news ran headlines declaring, "Elevator Enigma: Metropolis Grinds to a Halt in Stuck Elevator Incident!"

But amidst the chaos and confusion, there were moments of levity and laughter as the stranded passengers attempted to make the best of their situation. Some cracked jokes to lighten the mood, while others broke out into impromptu sing-alongs or started playing games to pass the time.

But the truth, as it turned out, was far simpler (and sillier) than anyone could have imagined. One day, as the occupants of the stuck elevator were finally rescued by a team of skilled technicians, they noticed something peculiar: perched atop the control panel was a mischievous pigeon, its feathers ruffled and its beady eyes gleaming with mischief.

It seemed that the pigeon, in a bid to add a bit of excitement to its mundane existence, had flown into the elevator shaft and inadvertently triggered the emergency stop button, bringing the elevator to a screeching halt and trapping its occupants inside.

From that day forward, Metropolis became known as the city that had a close encounter with the avian kind, a place where even the smallest of creatures could cause the biggest of headaches.

And so, as the stranded passengers bid farewell to the Great Stuck Elevator Incident and returned to their daily lives, they did so with a newfound appreciation for the unpredictability of city living and a story they would be telling for years to come.

The Sticky Situation: A Whimsical Tale of the Great Bubble Gum Wall Incident

In the quaint town of Gumdropville, where the streets were lined with candy-colored houses and the scent of sugar filled the air, there occurred an event that would go down in history as the Great Bubble Gum Wall Incident.

It all began one sunny afternoon, as the residents of Gumdropville gathered in the town square for the annual Bubble Gum Festival. The festival was a celebration of all things sweet and sticky, with games, contests, and of course, plenty of bubble gum to go around.

But as the festivities reached their peak and the residents indulged in their favorite chewy treat, disaster struck. A mischievous group of children, armed with handfuls of bubble gum and a sense of mischief, decided to see just how far they could stretch the limits of bubble gum creativity.

With giggles and grins, they began to stick their chewed gum to the side of a nearby building, fashioning it into intricate patterns and shapes that sparkled in the sunlight. What started as a playful prank soon escalated into a full-blown art installation, with the entire wall covered from top to bottom in a colorful mosaic of bubble gum.

Word of the bubble gum wall spread like wildfire through Gumdropville, drawing curious onlookers and concerned officials from far and wide. Soon, the streets were abuzz with whispers and speculation as the townsfolk debated the merits of the sticky spectacle.

The local news ran headlines declaring, "Sweet Surprise: Gumdropville's Great Bubble Gum Wall Incident Leaves Town in a Sticky Situation!"

But amidst the chaos and confusion, there were moments of levity and laughter as the residents marveled at the sheer audacity of the bubble gum artists. Some joked about the wall becoming a new tourist attraction, while others pondered the best way to clean up the sticky mess.

But the truth, as it turned out, was far simpler (and sillier) than anyone could have imagined. One day, as the residents of Gumdropville gathered to admire the bubble gum wall and ponder its fate, they noticed something peculiar: perched atop the highest point of the wall was a mischievous squirrel, its cheeks bulging with a mouthful of bubble gum.

It seemed that the squirrel, in a fit of playful curiosity, had decided to join in on the fun and contribute its sticky masterpiece to the wall. And while the residents may have been initially dismayed by the unexpected addition, they couldn't help but chuckle at the absurdity of it all.

From that day forward, Gumdropville became known as the town that had a close encounter of the chewy kind, a place where even the stickiest of situations could lead to laughter and camaraderie.

And so, as the residents bid farewell to the Great Bubble Gum Wall Incident and pondered its eventual fate, they did so with smiles on their faces and a newfound appreciation for the whimsy and wonder of life in Gumdropville.

The Twisted Tango: A Hilarious Tale of the Great "Twist" Dance-Off

In the lively town of Grooveville, where the streets were alive with the sound of music and the rhythm of dancing feet, there occurred an event that would go down in history as the Great "Twist" Dance-Off.

It all began one balmy evening, as the residents of Grooveville gathered in the town square for the annual dance competition. The atmosphere was electric with excitement as dancers of all ages and backgrounds prepared to showcase their moves and vie for the title of "Twist Champion."

But little did they know, they were about to encounter a twist of fate that would turn the competition on its head and leave the town laughing for years to come.

As the competition got underway, the dancers took to the floor with gusto, twirling and gyrating to the beat of the music with all the enthusiasm of seasoned pros. But then, just as the competition was reaching its peak, disaster struck.

With a sudden screech of feedback and a burst of static, the music cut out, leaving the dancers frozen in mid-twist and the crowd staring in disbelief. It seemed that the town's resident DJ had experienced a technical malfunction, bringing the dance-off to an unexpected halt.

But instead of letting the mishap dampen their spirits, the dancers seized upon the opportunity to showcase their creativity and improvisation skills. With a twinkle in their eyes and a spring in their step, they began to invent new twists and turns on the spot, transforming the dance-off into a spontaneous showcase of talent and ingenuity.

Word of the impromptu dance-off spread like wildfire through Grooveville, drawing curious onlookers and eager participants from far and wide. Soon, the streets were filled with laughter and applause as dancers of all ages joined in the fun, twisting and twirling with abandon as they improvised their way to dance-floor glory.

The local news ran headlines declaring, "Dance Disaster Turns into Delight: Grooveville's Great 'Twist' Dance-Off Leaves Town in Stitches!"

But amidst the laughter and applause, there were moments of genuine admiration as the dancers pushed the boundaries of creativity and expression. Some spun like whirligigs, while others wiggled and jiggled with all the grace of a bowl of gelatin.

But the true stars of the show were the town's youngest residents, who threw caution to the wind and danced with reckless abandon, their laughter echoing through the streets and their smiles lighting up the night.

From that day forward, Grooveville became known as the town that had a close encounter of the twisted kind, a place where even the simplest of mishaps could lead to laughter, camaraderie, and a whole lot of dancing.

And so, as the dancers bid farewell to the Great "Twist" Dance-Off and returned to their daily lives, they did so with a newfound appreciation for the joy of spontaneous creativity and the power of music to bring people together in laughter and harmony.

Woof Couture: The Whimsical Tale of the Space-Age Dog Fashion Show

In the bustling city of Pawsington, where the streets were filled with wagging tails and the bark of fashionistas echoed through the air, there occurred an event that would go down in history as the Space-Age Dog Fashion Show.

It all began on a sunny afternoon, as the residents of Pawsington gathered in the town square for a celebration of all things canine couture. The theme of the day was "Space Age Chic," and the dogs of Pawsington were ready to strut their stuff in the most out-of-this-world outfits imaginable.

As the fashion show got underway, the streets were transformed into a runway of intergalactic glamour, with dogs of all shapes and sizes parading down the catwalk in their space-themed ensembles. There were dogs dressed as astronauts, complete with helmets and space suits, and others adorned in glittering silver capes and futuristic goggles.

But amidst the glitz and glamor, there were moments of hilarity and whimsy as the dogs embraced the spirit of the occasion with gusto. Some pranced and pirouetted with all the grace of runway models, while others stumbled and tripped over their oversized costumes, much to the amusement of the crowd.

The local news ran headlines declaring, "Pawsington Goes Galactic: Space-Age Dog Fashion Show Leaves Town Howling with Laughter!"

But amidst the laughter and applause, there were moments of genuine admiration as the dogs showcased their creativity and individuality. Some had spent weeks crafting their costumes, while others had simply raided their owners' closets in search of the perfect space-age accessories.

But the true star of the show was a small pug named Cosmo, whose homemade rocket ship costume stole the hearts of the audience and earned him the title of "Best in Show." With his ears perked and his tail wagging, Cosmo pranced down the runway with all the confidence of a true space explorer, his owners beaming with pride by his side.

From that day forward, Pawsington became known as the city that had a close encounter with the canine kind, a place where even the most ordinary of pets could become fashion icons and bring joy to all who crossed their path.

And so, as the dogs of Pawsington bid farewell to the Space-Age Dog Fashion Show and returned to their lives of everyday adventure, they did so with a wag of their tails and a twinkle in their eyes, knowing that they had left an indelible mark on the world of fashion and brought smiles to the faces of all who witnessed their out-of-this-world style.

The Peanut Prank Pandemonium: A Nutty Tale That Had the Whole Campus Cracking Up

Once upon a time, on the sprawling campus of Nutty University, where the squirrels ruled the lawns and the trees whispered secrets in the breeze, there occurred a prank that would go down in history as the Peanut Prank Pandemonium.

It all started innocently enough when a mischievous group of students decided to play a harmless prank on their friends by scattering peanuts all over the campus grounds. Little did they know, their prank would spiral out of control and lead to a nutty chain of events that had the entire campus "peanut-ed."

As the students giggled and snickered, they hid behind bushes and trees, watching with glee as their unsuspecting classmates stumbled upon the peanuts and were left scratching their heads in confusion. But what started as a simple prank soon took on a life of its own, as the peanuts began to multiply and spread like wildfire, covering every inch of the campus in a sea of shells.

Word of the peanut prank spread like wildfire through Nutty University, drawing curious onlookers and concerned officials from far and wide.

Soon, the campus was abuzz with whispers and speculation as the students tried to unravel the mystery of the never-ending peanuts.

The local news ran headlines declaring, "Nutty University Goes Nuts: Peanut Prank Leaves Campus in Shells Shock!"

But amidst the chaos and confusion, there were moments of laughter and camaraderie as the students banded together to clean up the mess and restore order to their beloved campus. Some donned hazmat suits and gloves, while others armed themselves with brooms and dustpans, determined to rid the campus of its peanut problem once and for all.

But the truth, as it turned out, was far simpler (and sillier) than anyone could have imagined. One day, as the students were busy sweeping up the last of the peanuts, they noticed something peculiar: perched atop a nearby tree was a mischievous squirrel, its cheeks bulging with a mouthful of peanuts and its eyes twinkling with mischief.

It seemed that the squirrel, in a bid to add a bit of excitement to its mundane existence, had taken it upon itself to join in on the prank and spread peanuts all over the campus. And while the students may have been initially dismayed by the unexpected turn of events, they couldn't help but chuckle at the absurdity of it all.

From that day forward, Nutty University became known as the campus that had a close encounter with the nutty kind, a place where even the smallest of creatures could make a big impact on campus life.

And so, as the students bid farewell to the Peanut Prank Pandemonium and returned to their studies with a renewed sense of humor and camaraderie, they did so with a smile on their faces and a newfound appreciation for the nutty adventures that awaited them at Nutty University.

Disco Duck Mania: A Quacky Tale of the Great "Disco Duck" Craze

Once upon a time, in the groovy town of Funkytown, where the streets pulsed with rhythm and the beat of the disco ball lit up the night sky, there occurred a phenomenon that would go down in history as the Great "Disco Duck" Craze.

It all began one fateful night, as the residents of Funkytown gathered at the hottest disco club in town, "The Funky Feathers," to boogie the night away. The DJ, known for his funky beats and eclectic taste in music, decided to mix things up and play a quirky new song that had been making waves on the airwaves: "Disco Duck."

As the catchy tune filled the air and the dance floor came alive with pulsating energy, something miraculous happened. A lone duck, drawn by the irresistible rhythm of the music, waddled onto the dance floor and began to strut its stuff with all the confidence of a disco diva.

The sight of the duck grooving to the beat sent the crowd into a frenzy of excitement and laughter. They cheered and clapped as the duck spun and twirled, its feathers ruffled and its beak held high in a display of pure disco glory.

Word of the disco duck spread like wildfire through Funkytown, drawing curious onlookers and eager dancers from far and wide. Soon, "The Funky Feathers" was packed to the rafters with people eager to catch a glimpse of the legendary disco duck in action.

The local news ran headlines declaring, "Funky Feathers Frenzy: Disco Duck Takes Funkytown by Storm!"

But amidst the disco fever and excitement, there were moments of hilarity and whimsy as the residents of Funkytown embraced the quacky new dance craze with open arms. Some donned feathered boas and sparkling disco outfits, while others attempted to mimic the duck's signature moves with varying degrees of success.

But the true star of the show was the duck itself, who had unwittingly become the mascot of Funkytown's disco scene. With its infectious energy and undeniable charm, the disco duck inspired a whole new generation of dancers to shake their tail feathers and embrace the joy of dance.

From that day forward, Funkytown became known as the town that had a close encounter with the feathered kind, a place where even the most unlikely of creatures could become disco legends and bring joy to all who crossed their path.

And so, as the residents of Funkytown bid farewell to the Great "Disco Duck" Craze and returned to their daily lives with a renewed sense of fun and frivolity, they did so with a smile on their faces and a disco beat in their hearts, knowing that they had been part of something truly quack-tactic.

The Hot Dog Havoc: A Hilarious Tale of the Epic Eating Contest Mishap

In the lively town of Bellyville, where the scent of sizzling sausages filled the air and the sound of stomachs growling echoed through the streets, there occurred an event that would go down in history as the Hot Dog Havoc: the annual Hot Dog Eating Contest.

It all began one sunny afternoon, as the residents of Bellyville gathered in the town square for the highly anticipated event. The competition was fierce, with contenders from all corners of the town vying for the title of Hot Dog Eating Champion and the coveted Golden Mustard Bottle trophy.

As the contestants took their places at the long table piled high with hot dogs, the crowd cheered and jeered, egging them on to eat as many wieners as humanly possible in the allotted time. But little did they know, they were about to witness a mishap of epic proportions that would leave them rolling with laughter.

As the clock ticked down and the contestants dove headfirst into their piles of hot dogs, it quickly became apparent that one competitor, a bumbling baker named Benny, had bitten off more than he could chew.

With each hot dog he attempted to swallow, another seemed to pop right back up, leaving him in a comical battle of wits with the unruly sausages.

The crowd erupted into fits of laughter as Benny's face turned red with exertion and his cheeks bulged with half-eaten hot dogs. He frantically dunked his buns in water and gulped down mouthfuls of soda in a desperate bid to make room for more, but to no avail.

The local news ran headlines declaring, "Bellyville's Belly-Buster: Hilarious Hot Dog Eating Contest Mishap Leaves Town in Stitches!"

But amidst the laughter and chaos, there were moments of genuine admiration as Benny refused to give up, even in the face of certain defeat. With tears of laughter streaming down their faces, the crowd cheered him on as he valiantly soldiered on, determined to finish what he had started.

But the true hero of the day was not Benny, nor any of the other contestants. It was the humble hot dog itself, which had unwittingly become the star of the show and brought joy and laughter to all who witnessed its role in the hilarious mishap.

From that day forward, Bellyville became known as the town that had a close encounter of the culinary kind, a place where even the simplest of foods could become the catalyst for laughter and camaraderie.

And so, as Benny bid farewell to the Hot Dog Havoc and returned to his bakery with a belly full of wieners and a smile on his face, he did so with a newfound appreciation for the joy of laughter and the power of a good old-fashioned hot dog eating contest gone hilariously awry.

The Melodic Mischief of the Singing Goldfish: A Fishy Tale

In the cozy town of Harmony Bay, where the gentle lapping of waves against the shore provided a soothing soundtrack to everyday life, there occurred an event that would go down in history as the Unlikely Case of the Singing Goldfish.

It all started one serene afternoon, as the residents of Harmony Bay went about their daily routines, blissfully unaware of the musical marvel that was about to unfold. In the quiet confines of Mrs. Smith's living room, a curious scene was unfolding.

As Mrs. Smith sat down at her piano to practice her scales, she noticed something peculiar: her pet goldfish, named Mozart, swimming circles in its bowl and emitting a series of melodious chirps. At first, Mrs. Smith dismissed it as a figment of her imagination, but as the notes grew louder and more distinct, she realized that her fish was indeed singing along to her music!

Word of the singing goldfish spread like wildfire through Harmony Bay, drawing curious onlookers and eager music enthusiasts from far and wide. Soon, Mrs. Smith's living room was transformed into an impromptu concert hall, with crowds gathering outside her window to catch a glimpse of the musical marvel within.

The local news ran headlines declaring, "Harmony Bay's Fishy Phenomenon: Singing Goldfish Leaves Town Speechless!"

But amidst the awe and wonder, there were moments of hilarity and whimsy as the residents of Harmony Bay tried to wrap their heads around the bizarre spectacle. Some joked about forming a fish choir, while others speculated on the secret to Mozart's musical talents.

But the true star of the show was Mozart himself, who had unwittingly become the town's newest sensation. With each chirp and trill, he captivated audiences with his unique brand of underwater opera, leaving them in stitches of laughter and applause.

From that day forward, Harmony Bay became known as the town that had a close encounter of the aquatic kind, a place where even the most unlikely of creatures could become musical prodigies and bring joy to all who listened.

And so, as Mrs. Smith bid farewell to her singing goldfish and returned to her daily routines with a newfound appreciation for the wonders of the natural world, she did so with a smile on her face and a song in her heart, knowing that she had been part of something truly fish-macular.

The Rubber Chicken Riot: A Feather-Ruffling Fiasco

In the whimsical town of Clucksville, where the streets were lined with feathers and the clucking of chickens filled the air, there occurred an event that would go down in history as the Great Rubber Chicken Rebellion.

It all started one sunny day, as the residents of Clucksville gathered for the annual poultry parade, a celebration of all things feathered and fabulous. Among the floats and festivities, a group of mischievous pranksters decided to shake things up by introducing a new addition to the parade: rubber chickens.

At first, the sight of rubber chickens bobbing along the parade route elicited chuckles and smiles from the crowd. But as more and more rubber chickens made their appearance, the laughter turned to confusion, and then to outrage.

The local chickens, proud residents of Clucksville, were incensed by the mockery of their feathered brethren. They squawked and flapped their wings in protest, demanding that the rubber chickens be banished from the parade and their honor restored.

Word of the rubber chicken rebellion spread like wildfire through Clucksville, drawing curious onlookers and concerned officials from far and wide. Soon, the streets were filled with clucking and chaos as the town descended into a feather-ruffling fiasco.

The local news ran headlines declaring, "Clucksville in Crisis: Rubber Chicken Rebellion Ruffles Feathers!"

But amidst the chaos and confusion, there were moments of hilarity and whimsy as the townsfolk tried to make sense of the absurd situation. Some attempted to negotiate a truce between the feuding factions, while others simply sat back and enjoyed the spectacle.

But the true heroes of the day were the rubber chickens themselves, who had unwittingly sparked a revolution and brought laughter and joy to the residents of Clucksville. With each squawk and squeak, they reminded everyone that sometimes, it's okay to embrace the absurd and let loose a little.

From that day forward, Clucksville became known as the town that had a close encounter with the rubbery kind, a place where even the most unlikely of objects could spark a revolution and bring a smile to the faces of all who witnessed it.

And so, as the residents of Clucksville bid farewell to the Great Rubber Chicken Rebellion and returned to their daily lives with a newfound appreciation for the power of laughter, they did so with a cluck and a chuckle, knowing that they had been part of something truly egg-cellent.

The Lively Llama Limousine Adventure: A Tale of Llamas and Laughter

In the quaint town of Llamaville, where the hills were alive with the sound of bleating and the streets were lined with woolly wonders, there occurred an event that would go down in history as the Legendary Llama Limo Ride.

It all started one sunny day, as the residents of Llamaville gathered for the annual llama festival, a celebration of all things llama-related. Among the festivities was a special treat for the townsfolk: a llama-themed limousine ride through the scenic countryside.

As the townsfolk lined up for their turn to hop aboard the llama limo, excitement filled the air. But little did they know, their llama-filled adventure was about to take a hilarious turn.

As the limousine set off down the winding roads, the passengers were treated to a sight like no other: llamas, decked out in their finest attire, lounging regally in the back of the limo as they sipped on carrot martinis and nibbled on alfalfa hors d'oeuvres.

The local news ran headlines declaring, "Llama Limousine Lunacy: Llamaville Residents Take a Ride on the Wild Side!"

But amidst the laughter and excitement, there were moments of sheer absurdity as the llamas embraced their newfound status as VIPs. Some struck poses for the cameras, while others attempted to give interviews in their best llama language, much to the amusement of the passengers.

But the true stars of the show were the llamas themselves, who had unwittingly become the toast of Llamaville with their unforgettable limousine adventure. With each graceful swish of their tails and each dignified bleat, they reminded everyone that sometimes, the most unlikely of creatures can steal the show.

From that day forward, Llamaville became known as the town that had a close encounter with the llama kind, a place where even the most ordinary of events could become an unforgettable adventure.

And so, as the residents of Llamaville bid farewell to their legendary llama limo ride and returned to their daily lives with a smile on their faces and a chuckles in their hearts, they did so with a newfound appreciation for the magic of llamas and the joy they bring to the world around them.

The Hilarious Horseplay: A Tale of the Pantomime Horse Parade Prank

In the lively town of Jesterfield, where laughter filled the air and silliness was celebrated with gusto, there occurred an event that would go down in history as the Pantomime Horse Parade Prank.

It all started one sunny day, as the residents of Jesterfield gathered for their annual parade, a spectacle of whimsy and merriment. Among the floats and performers, a group of mischievous pranksters had hatched a plan to add a bit of absurdity to the proceedings: they would stage a pantomime horse parade prank like no other.

As the parade wound its way through the streets of Jesterfield, spectators cheered and waved as the floats passed by. But then, to their astonishment, they spotted something truly bizarre: a procession of pantomime horses, each consisting of two people dressed in elaborate horse costumes.

The local news ran headlines declaring, "Jesterfield's Jocular Jape: Pantomime Horse Parade Prank Leaves Town in Stitches!"

But amidst the laughter and confusion, there were moments of sheer absurdity as the pantomime horses pranced and danced their way through the streets. Some attempted to gallop in unison, while others engaged in playful horseplay, much to the amusement of the crowd.

But the true stars of the show were the pranksters themselves, who had unwittingly become the talk of the town with their outrageous antics. With each exaggerated trot and exaggerated whinny, they reminded everyone that sometimes, the best way to spread joy is to embrace the absurd.

From that day forward, Jesterfield became known as the town that had a close encounter of the equine kind, a place where even the most ordinary of parades could become an unforgettable spectacle of silliness.

And so, as the residents of Jesterfield bid farewell to the Pantomime Horse Parade Prank and returned to their daily lives with a smile on their faces and a chuckles in their hearts, they did so with a newfound appreciation for the joy of laughter and the power of a good old-fashioned prank.

Granny's Groovy Glide: The Tale of the Unexpected Skateboarding Granny

In the quaint neighborhood of Sunnydale, where the streets were lined with cozy cottages and the scent of freshly baked cookies wafted through the air, there lived a grandmother named Mildred. Mildred was known throughout the neighborhood for her warm smile, her delicious pies, and her love of all things traditional.

But little did the residents of Sunnydale know, Mildred had a secret passion that would soon take the neighborhood by storm: skateboarding.

It all started one sunny afternoon, as Mildred sat on her porch, knitting a cozy sweater for her grandson. As she watched the neighborhood kids skateboarding down the street, she couldn't help but feel a twinge of curiosity.

With a mischievous glint in her eye, Mildred decided to give skateboarding a try. She dusted off an old skateboard she had found in the attic and gingerly stepped onto it, wobbling uncertainly at first.

But to her surprise, Mildred found herself gaining confidence with each push of her foot. Before long, she was gliding down the street with all the grace and poise of a seasoned pro, her silver hair trailing behind her like a superhero's cape.

The local news ran headlines declaring, "Sunnydale's Skateboarding Sensation: Granny Shreds the Streets!"

But amidst the laughter and applause, there were moments of sheer disbelief as the residents of Sunnydale watched Mildred perform daring tricks and stunts that defied her age. Some cheered her on from the sidelines, while others scrambled to capture her incredible feats on camera.

But the true star of the show was Mildred herself, who had unwittingly become the talk of the town with her unexpected skateboarding skills. With each twist and turn, she reminded everyone that age is just a number and that it's never too late to try something new.

From that day forward, Sunnydale became known as the neighborhood that had a close encounter with the granny kind, a place where even the most unlikely of residents could surprise and inspire with their hidden talents.

And so, as Mildred bid farewell to her newfound fame and returned to her knitting with a smile on her face and a sense of pride in her heart, she did so knowing that she had shown the world that you're never too old to embrace your inner skateboarder and glide through life with style and grace.

Let's go Back To the 70's

The Rock Stars: A Rockin' Tale of the Great Pet Rock Craze

Once upon a time, in the bustling town of Pebbleville, where the streets were paved with stones and the rocks outnumbered the residents, there occurred an event that would go down in history as the Great Pet Rock Craze.

It all began on a lazy afternoon, as the residents of Pebbleville stumbled upon a curious sight: a group of friends, gathered in the town square, admiring their newest companions - pet rocks. These rocks, adorned with googly eyes and painted smiles, had captured the hearts of the townsfolk in an instant.

As word of the pet rock craze spread like wildfire through Pebbleville, the town was transformed into a rockin' paradise. Everywhere you looked, people were proudly displaying their pet rocks, giving them names, and even taking them for walks on makeshift leashes.

The local news ran headlines declaring, "Pebbleville's Rock Stars: The Great Pet Rock Craze Rocks the Town!"

But amidst the laughter and excitement, there were moments of sheer absurdity as the residents of Pebbleville embraced their newfound rock companions with gusto. Some held pet rock fashion shows, while others organized rock-themed parties and parades.

But the true stars of the show were the pet rocks themselves, who had unwittingly become the talk of the town with their silent charm and unwavering loyalty. With each painted smile and each googly-eyed gaze, they reminded everyone that sometimes, the simplest things in life can bring the greatest joy.

From that day forward, Pebbleville became known as the town that had a close encounter with the rocky kind, a place where even the most ordinary of objects could become cherished companions and bring laughter and happiness to all who embraced them.

And so, as the residents of Pebbleville bid farewell to the Great Pet Rock Craze and returned to their daily lives with a smile on their faces and a rock in their pockets, they did so with a newfound appreciation for the whimsy and wonder of life in their rockin' little town.

The Disco Debacle: A Hilarious Tale of the "Disco Sucks" Rally

Once upon a time, in the vibrant city of Grooveburg, where the disco ball spun and the dance floors thumped with the beat of funky tunes, there occurred an event that would go down in history as the "Disco Sucks" Rally.

It all began on a balmy summer evening, as a group of disgruntled rock 'n' roll enthusiasts gathered in the town square to protest the rising popularity of disco music. Armed with signs bearing slogans like "Disco Is a No-Go" and "Rock 'n' Roll Forever," they were determined to make their voices heard.

As the rally kicked off, the protesters marched through the streets of Grooveburg, chanting anti-disco slogans and waving their banners high. But little did they know, their protest was about to take an unexpected turn.

Just as the rally reached its peak, a group of disco dancers emerged from a nearby nightclub, their glittering costumes and funky dance moves in stark contrast to the protesters' somber attire. With a twirl and a spin, they joined the rally, adding a splash of disco flair to the proceedings.

The local news ran headlines declaring, "Grooveburg's Disco Dilemma: 'Disco Sucks' Rally Turns into a Dance Party!"

But amidst the confusion and chaos, there were moments of sheer hilarity as the protesters found themselves caught up in the infectious energy of the disco dancers. Some attempted to resist the urge to boogie, while others threw caution to the wind and embraced the disco fever with open arms.

But the true stars of the show were the disco dancers themselves, who had unwittingly turned the "Disco Sucks" Rally into an impromptu dance party that had the whole town laughing and grooving along.

From that day forward, Grooveburg became known as the city that had a close encounter of the disco kind, a place where even the most unlikely of events could turn into a hilarious and unforgettable spectacle.

And so, as the protesters and disco dancers bid farewell to the "Disco Sucks" Rally and returned to their daily lives with a smile on their faces and a disco beat in their hearts, they did so knowing that they had been part of something truly groovy.

The Fizzy Fiasco: A Comical Tale of the Infamous "Coke" Hoax

In the bustling town of Bubblesville, where soda fizzed and laughter bubbled, there occurred an event that would go down in history as the Infamous "Coke" Hoax.

It all began one sunny day, as a mischievous group of friends decided to play a prank on the unsuspecting residents of Bubblesville. Armed with bottles of plain sparkling water and a few drops of food coloring, they set out to create their version of the world-famous soda: Coca-Cola.

As the pranksters distributed their homemade "Coke" to unsuspecting passersby, the reactions were priceless. Some sipped cautiously, only to recoil in confusion at the lack of sweetness. Others took a gulp and immediately spat it out, convinced that they had been tricked.

The local news ran headlines declaring, "Bubblesville's Bubbly Blunder: Infamous 'Coke' Hoax Leaves Town in Bubbles!"

But amidst the chaos and confusion, there were moments of sheer hilarity as the residents of Bubblesville attempted to make sense of the fizzy fiasco. Some laughed it off as a harmless prank, while others shook their heads in disbelief at the audacity of the pranksters.

But the true stars of the show were the pranksters themselves, who had unwittingly turned Bubblesville into a laughingstock with their comical caper. With each sip and each smirk, they reminded everyone that sometimes, the best way to spread joy is to embrace the absurd.

From that day forward, Bubblesville became known as the town that had a close encounter of the fizzy kind, a place where even the most ordinary of beverages could become the catalyst for laughter and merriment.

And so, as the residents of Bubblesville bid farewell to the Infamous "Coke" Hoax and returned to their daily lives with a smile on their faces and a chuckle in their hearts, they did so knowing that they had been part of something truly fizzy and fun.

The Grinning Epidemic: A Whimsical Tale of the Great "Smile Face" Craze

Once upon a time, in the cheerful town of Joyville, where laughter echoed through the streets and happiness was contagious, there occurred an event that would go down in history as the Great "Smile Face" Craze.

It all started innocently enough, with a simple doodle of a smiling face drawn on a piece of paper by a playful child. Little did they know, their creation would soon spread like wildfire, bringing smiles to the faces of everyone it touched.

As the "smile face" doodle made its way through Joyville, it seemed to take on a life of its own. People began to incorporate the smiling face into everything they did, from decorating their homes to wearing it on their clothing. Soon, the entire town was awash with grinning faces, each one brighter and more infectious than the last.

The local news ran headlines declaring, "Joyville's Jovial Jamboree: The Great 'Smile Face' Craze Spreads Like Wildfire!"

But amidst the laughter and joy, there were moments of sheer absurdity as the residents of Joyville embraced the craze with gusto. Some painted smile faces on their cars, while others formed smile face clubs and held meetings to discuss their love of all things cheerful.

But the true star of the show was the smile face itself, which had unwittingly become the symbol of Joyville's infectious spirit. With each grin and each giggle, it reminded everyone that sometimes, a simple smile is all it takes to brighten someone's day.

From that day forward, Joyville became known as the town that had a close encounter with the smiley kind, a place where even the smallest of gestures could spread happiness far and wide.

And so, as the residents of Joyville bid farewell to the Great "Smile Face" Craze and returned to their daily lives with a smile on their faces and a twinkle in their eyes, they did so knowing that they had been part of something truly whimsical and wonderful.

The Wacky Races: A Zany Tale of Legendary Laughter

Once upon a time, in the quirky town of Goofytown, where laughter was the currency and silliness was celebrated, there occurred an event that would go down in history as the Legendary "Wacky Races."

It all started one bright and sunny day, as the residents of Goofytown gathered at the starting line for the most outrageous race the town had ever seen. The air was electric with excitement as a motley crew of competitors revved their engines and prepared for the wackiest race of their lives.

The race featured an eclectic mix of vehicles, from flying saucers to rocket-powered roller skates, each one more absurd than the last. As the starting flag waved, the competitors raced off into the wild unknown, leaving a trail of chaos and laughter in their wake.

The local news ran headlines declaring, "Goofytown's Gigglefest: Legendary 'Wacky Races' Leaves Town in Stitches!"

But amidst the chaos and hilarity, there were moments of sheer madness as the racers encountered obstacles and challenges that seemed straight out of a cartoon. Some navigated through a maze of giant rubber ducks, while others dodged flying pies and banana peels with expert precision.

But the true stars of the show were the racers themselves, who had unwittingly become the talk of the town with their outrageous antics and daring maneuvers. With each lap and each leap, they reminded everyone that sometimes, the best way to win a race is to embrace the absurd and let loose a little.

From that day forward, Goofytown became known as the town that had a close encounter with the wacky kind, a place where even the most ordinary of events could become an unforgettable spectacle of silliness and laughter.

And so, as the racers bid farewell to the Legendary "Wacky Races" and returned to their daily lives with a smile on their faces and a chuckle in their hearts, they did so knowing that they had been part of something truly legendary and wonderfully wacky.

The Bovine Bungle: A Moo-ving Tale of the Case of the Stolen Cow Mascot

In the quaint town of Dairyville, where the air was sweet with the scent of fresh milk and the cows roamed contentedly in the fields, there occurred an event that would go down in history as the Case of the Stolen Cow Mascot.

It all began on a sunny morning, as the residents of Dairyville awoke to find their beloved cow mascot, Bessie, missing from her usual spot in front of the local dairy farm. Bessie, a life-sized fiberglass cow with a jovial smile and a friendly wave, had long been a symbol of pride for the town.

As news of Bessie's disappearance spread like wildfire through Dairyville, the townsfolk were overcome with shock and disbelief. How could someone steal a cow, let alone a giant fiberglass one?

The local news ran headlines declaring, "Dairyville's Dilemma: Case of the Stolen Cow Mascot Leaves Town in Udder Disbelief!"

But amidst the confusion and chaos, there were moments of sheer absurdity as the residents of Dairyville attempted to unravel the mystery of Bessie's disappearance. Some speculated that she had been abducted by aliens, while others pointed fingers at rival towns in a dairy-themed feud.

But the true heroes of the story were a group of plucky youngsters, led by a determined young girl named Daisy, who had unwittingly stumbled upon a clue that would crack the case wide open. While exploring the outskirts of town, they stumbled upon Bessie, hidden away in a barn and adorned with a makeshift disguise of sunglasses and a cowboy hat.

With a giggle and a grin, Daisy and her friends brought Bessie back to Dairyville, where she was greeted with cheers and applause from the relieved townsfolk. As it turned out, Bessie had been taken as a prank by a group of mischievous teenagers from a neighboring town, who had intended to use her as a prop in their cow-themed festivities.

From that day forward, Dairyville became known as the town that had a close encounter with the bovine kind, a place where even the most absurd of mysteries could be solved with a little laughter and a lot of determination.

And so, as the residents of Dairyville bid farewell to the Case of the Stolen Cow Mascot and returned to their daily lives with a smile on their faces and a cow-shaped mascot in their hearts, they did so knowing that they had been part of a truly moo-ving adventure.

The Sweet Shambles: A Whimsical Tale of The Great "Candy Necklace" Incident

Once upon a time, in the colorful town of Sugartown, where candy-coated the streets and sugar filled the air, there occurred an event that would go down in history as The Great "Candy Necklace" Incident.

It all began on a sunny day, as the residents of Sugartown gathered for the annual candy festival, a celebration of all things sweet and sugary. Among the festivities was a contest to create the longest candy necklace the town had ever seen.

As the contestants eagerly strung together colorful candies, excitement filled the air. But little did they know, their sweet creation was about to take an unexpected turn.

Just as the final pieces of candy were added to the necklace, disaster struck. With a loud snap, the weight of the candies proved too much for the string to bear, and the entire necklace came crashing down in a sticky heap.

The local news ran headlines declaring, "Sugartown's Sticky Situation: The Great 'Candy Necklace' Incident Leaves Town in a Sugar-Coated Mess!"

But amidst the chaos and commotion, there were moments of sheer hilarity as the residents of Sugartown attempted to salvage what was left of the candy necklace. Some dove headfirst into the pile of candies, while others simply shrugged and laughed at the absurdity of it all.

But the true heroes of the day were a group of resourceful children, who had unwittingly stumbled upon a solution to the sticky situation. With a little ingenuity and a lot of laughter, they transformed the fallen candy necklace into a giant candy sculpture that delighted the entire town.

From that day forward, Sugartown became known as the town that had a close encounter with the sugary kind, a place where even the stickiest of situations could be turned into a sweet success with a little creativity and a lot of laughter.

And so, as the residents of Sugartown bid farewell to The Great "Candy Necklace" Incident and returned to their daily lives with a smile on their faces and a sugar rush in their hearts, they did so knowing that they had been part of a truly whimsical and wonderful adventure.

The Clucking Comedy: A Feather-Ruffling Tale of The "Funky Chicken" Dance-Off

In the lively town of Featherland, where roosters crowed and hens clucked to the beat of the day, there occurred an event that would go down in history as The "Funky Chicken" Dance-Off.

It all started one sunny afternoon, as the residents of Featherland gathered in the town square for a day of festivities. Among the various competitions and activities, one stood out from the rest: The "Funky Chicken" Dance-Off.

As the music started to play, contestants of all shapes and sizes flapped their wings and strutted their stuff in a hilarious display of chicken-inspired dance moves. From the classic wing flaps to the funky chicken shuffle, there was no shortage of laughter and amusement.

The local news ran headlines declaring, "Featherland's Feather-Ruffling Fiasco: The "Funky Chicken" Dance-Off Leaves Town in Stitches!"

But amidst the clucking and chaos, there were moments of sheer absurdity as the contestants vied for the title of Funkiest Chicken in Featherland. Some attempted daring acrobatics, while others simply embraced the chicken spirit and let loose with wild abandon.

But the true star of the show was a plucky little chick named Cluckers, who had unwittingly stolen the spotlight with his outrageous dance moves and infectious enthusiasm. With each shake of his tail feathers and each squawk of delight, he had the entire town cheering him on.

From that day forward, Featherland became known as the town that had a close encounter with the feathered kind, a place where even the silliest of competitions could bring joy and laughter to all who participated.

And so, as the residents of Featherland bid farewell to The "Funky Chicken" Dance-Off and returned to their daily lives with a smile on their faces and a cluck in their hearts, they did so knowing that they had been part of a truly clucking good time.

The Peculiar Poodle Puzzle: A Hilarious Tale of the Missing "Poodle"

In the quaint neighborhood of Woofington, where the streets were lined with doghouses and the air was filled with barks and wagging tails, there occurred an event that would go down in history as The Case of the Missing "Poodle."

It all began one sunny afternoon, as the residents of Woofington gathered in the park for a canine carnival. Among the various attractions and activities, one stood out from the rest: a doggy fashion show featuring Woofington's most fashionable pooches.

As the fashion show kicked off with a parade of pampered pups strutting their stuff on the runway, there was one notable absence:

Priscilla, the prized poodle of Mrs. Fluffybottom. Priscilla, a fluffy white poodle with a penchant for pearls, was nowhere to be found.

The local news ran headlines declaring, "Woofington's Woeful Whodunit: The Case of the Missing 'Poodle' Leaves Town in a Tailspin!"

But amidst the confusion and commotion, there were moments of sheer hilarity as the residents of Woofington attempted to solve the mystery of Priscilla's disappearance. Some sniffed out clues with their keen noses, while others chased their tails in circles, convinced they were hot on the trail.

But the true heroes of the day were a group of mischievous squirrels, who had unwittingly squirreled away Priscilla in their treehouse hideout. With a twinkle in their eyes and a mischievous chitter, they watched from above as the residents of Woofington scurried about in search of the missing poodle.

From that day forward, Woofington became known as the town that had a close encounter with the furry kind, a place where even the most peculiar of mysteries could be solved with a little laughter and a lot of wagging tails.

And so, as the residents of Woofington bid farewell to The Case of the Missing "Poodle" and returned to their daily lives with a smile on their faces and a wag in their tails, they did so knowing that they had been part of a truly doggone funny adventure.

The Leisure Suit Lunacy: A Silly Tale of the Great "Leisure Suit" Fad

Once upon a time, in the groovy town of Funkytown, where disco balls glittered and funk music filled the air, there occurred an event that would go down in history as The Great "Leisure Suit" Fad.

It all started one sunny day, as a fashion craze swept through Funkytown like wildfire. The streets were suddenly filled with people sporting flamboyant leisure suits in vibrant colors and flashy patterns. From bright orange to electric blue, there was no shortage of eye-catching ensembles.

The local news ran headlines declaring, "Funkytown's Funky Fad: The Great 'Leisure Suit' Craze Takes Town by Storm!"

But amidst the excitement and laughter, there were moments of sheer absurdity as the residents of Funkytown embraced the leisure suit trend with gusto. Some strutted down the streets with exaggerated swagger, while others attempted to perfect the iconic disco dance moves that had become synonymous with the era.

But the true stars of the show were a group of eccentric characters known as the Leisure Suit Brigade, who had unwittingly become the darlings of Funkytown with their outlandish fashion choices and larger-than-life personalities. With each polyester-clad strut and each flashy accessory, they brought joy and laughter to all who crossed their path.

From that day forward, Funkytown became known as the town that had a close encounter of the funky kind, a place where even the most outrageous of fashion trends could bring people together in laughter and camaraderie.

And so, as the residents of Funkytown bid farewell to The Great "Leisure Suit" Fad and returned to their daily lives with a smiles on their faces and boogies in their steps, they did so knowing that they had been part of a truly groovy and hilarious adventure.

Disco Demolition Delirium: A Comical Tale of "Disco Demolition" Night

Once upon a time, in the bustling city of Boogieville, where disco balls sparkled and dance floors thumped with the beat of funky tunes, there occurred an event that would go down in history as Disco Demolition Night.

It all started on a hot summer evening, as the residents of Boogieville gathered at the local baseball stadium for a promotional event like no other. The plan was simple: attendees could bring their disco records and, in exchange, receive discounted admission to the game.

But little did anyone know, the event would soon spiral into chaos of comedic proportions.

As the stadium filled, a sense of excitement filled the air. But as the night went on, it became clear that things were about to take a turn for the absurd.

The local news ran headlines declaring, "Boogieville's Bizarre Bash: Disco Demolition Night Descends into Delirium!"

But amidst the chaos and confusion, there were moments of sheer hilarity as the residents of Boogieville attempted to make sense of the madness. Some danced on the field with reckless abandon, while others attempted to catch flying vinyl records with oversized mitts.

But the true stars of the show were a group of disco-loving fans, who had unwittingly become the heroes of Disco Demolition Night with their outrageous antics and infectious enthusiasm. With each vinyl record smashed and each disco ball destroyed, they brought laughter and joy to all who witnessed their antics.

From that day forward, Boogieville became known as the city that had a close encounter of the disco kind, a place where even the most unlikely of events could bring people together in laughter and camaraderie.

And so, as the residents of Boogieville bid farewell to Disco Demolition Night and returned to their daily lives with a smile on their faces and a boogie in their step, they did so knowing that they had been part of a truly groovy and hilarious adventure.

The Doughnut Dilemma: A Whimsical Tale of the Missing Giant Doughnut

In the charming town of Sweetville, where the aroma of freshly baked treats filled the air and sugar-coated the streets, there occurred an event that would go down in history as The Case of the Missing Giant Doughnut.

It all began one bright morning, as the residents of Sweetville awoke to find their beloved landmark, the Giant Doughnut, missing from its usual spot in the town square. The Giant Doughnut, a towering confectionery masterpiece, had long been a source of pride for the town.

As news of the doughnut's disappearance spread like frosting, the townsfolk were overcome with shock and disbelief. How could someone steal a doughnut the size of a house?

The local news ran headlines declaring, "Sweetville's Sweet Sensation: The Case of the Missing Giant Doughnut Leaves Town in a Sticky Situation!"

But amidst the confusion and commotion, there were moments of sheer hilarity as the residents of Sweetville attempted to solve the mystery. Some searched high and low, while others followed a trail of sprinkles and icing crumbs in search of clues.

But the true heroes of the day were a group of mischievous squirrels, who had unwittingly squirreled away the Giant Doughnut to their treehouse hideout. With a twinkle in their eyes and a mouthful of sugary delight, they watched from above as the residents of Sweetville scurried about in search of the missing doughnut.

From that day forward, Sweetville became known as the town that had a close encounter with the sugary kind, a place where even the most peculiar of mysteries could be solved with a little laughter and a lot of creativity.

And so, as the residents of Sweetville bid farewell to The Case of the Missing Giant Doughnut and returned to their daily lives with a smile on their faces and a sprinkle in their steps, they did so knowing that they had been part of a truly sweet and whimsical adventure.

The Rubber Chicken Revelry: A Hilarious Tale of the Great "Rubber Chicken" Parade

In the quirky town of Quirktown, where laughter echoed through the streets and silliness was celebrated, there occurred an event that would go down in history as The Great "Rubber Chicken" Parade.

It all started on a sunny day, as the residents of Quirktown gathered in the town square for a parade like no other. Instead of floats and marching bands, the parade featured a procession of people carrying rubber chickens of all shapes and sizes.

The rubber chickens, with their silly expressions and floppy bodies, quickly became the stars of the show. From the classic yellow chickens to the rainbow-colored ones, there was no shortage of laughter and amusement.

The local news ran headlines declaring, "Quirktown's Quirky Quack-fest: The Great 'Rubber Chicken' Parade Leaves Town in Stitches!"

But amidst the laughter and chaos, there were moments of sheer absurdity as the residents of Quirktown embraced the rubber chicken craze with gusto. Some twirled their chickens like batons, while others attempted to balance them on their heads or toss them high into the air.

But the true heroes of the day were a group of eccentric characters known as the Rubber Chicken Brigade, who had unwittingly become the darlings of Quirktown with their outlandish antics and larger-than-life personalities. With each rubbery squawk and each floppy waddle, they brought joy and laughter to all who crossed their path.

From that day forward, Quirktown became known as the town that had a close encounter of the rubbery kind, a place where even the silliest of parades could bring people together in laughter and camaraderie.

And so, as the residents of Quirktown bid farewell to The Great "Rubber Chicken" Parade and returned to their daily lives with a smile on their faces and rubber chicken in their hearts, they did so knowing that they had been part of a truly quack-tastic and hilarious adventure.

The Cheeky Craze: A Whimsical Tale of the "Mooning" Fad

Once upon a time, in the lively town of Cheeksville, where laughter echoed through the streets and mischief was celebrated, there occurred an event that would go down in history as The "Mooning" Craze.

It all started innocently enough, with a playful prank pulled by a group of mischievous teenagers. One moonlit night, they decided to bare their bottoms to pass cars from the safety of their backyard. Little did they know, their antics would spark a craze that would sweep through the town like wildfire.

As word of the prank spread, more and more people joined in on the fun. Soon, "mooning" became the talk of the town, with residents of all ages dropping trou and showing their backsides to anyone who dared to look.

The local news ran headlines declaring, "Cheeksville's Cheeky Shenanigans: The 'Mooning' Craze Leaves Town Blushing!"

But amidst the laughter and chaos, there were moments of sheer absurdity as the residents of Cheeksville embraced the craze with gusto. Some mooned from the rooftops, while others organized mooning flash mobs in the town square.

But the true stars of the show were a group of elderly ladies known as the "Mooning Grannies," who had unwittingly become the darlings of Cheeksville with their daring displays of cheekiness. With each wobbly moon and each infectious giggle, they brought joy and laughter to all who witnessed their antics.

From that day forward, Cheeksville became known as the town that had a close encounter with the cheeky kind, a place where even the most outrageous of fads could bring people together in laughter and camaraderie.

And so, as the residents of Cheeksville bid farewell to The "Mooning" Craze and returned to their daily lives with a smiles on their faces and chuckles in their hearts, they did so knowing that they had been part of a truly cheeky and hilarious adventure.

The Silly String Showdown: A Wacky Tale of the Great "Silly String" War

In the bustling town of Whimsyville, where laughter was the language and silliness was celebrated, there occurred an event that would go down in history as The Great "Silly String" War.

It all began on a sunny day, as the residents of Whimsyville gathered for the annual carnival. Among the games and rides, there was one attraction that stood out from the rest: a booth selling cans of silly string in every color of the rainbow.

As the day wore on and the cans of silly string flew off the shelves, it became clear that a battle was brewing. Soon, the streets of Whimsyville were filled with people armed with cans of silly string, ready to engage in the silliest of skirmishes.

The local news ran headlines declaring, "Whimsyville's Wacky War: The Great 'Silly String' Showdown Leaves Town in Stitches!"

But amidst the chaos and commotion, there were moments of sheer hilarity as the residents of Whimsyville engaged in the silliest of battles. Some sprayed their friends and neighbors with streams of silly string, while others attempted to create intricate patterns in the air with their cans.

But the true heroes of the day were a group of children, who had unwittingly become the leaders of the Silly String Brigade with their boundless energy and infectious laughter. With each squirt and each squeal of delight, they brought joy and laughter to all who joined in the fun.

From that day forward, Whimsyville became known as the town that had a close encounter of the silly kind, a place where even the most absurd of battles could bring people together in laughter and camaraderie.

And so, as the residents of Whimsyville bid farewell to The Great "Silly String" War and returned to their daily lives with a smile on their faces and a can of silly string in their hearts, they did so knowing that they had been part of a truly wacky and wonderful adventure.

The Sign Snafu: A Whimsical Tale of the Stolen Street Sign

In the quaint town of Quirktown, where the streets twisted and turned like a labyrinth and laughter echoed through the cobblestone alleys, there occurred an event that would go down in history as The Case of the Stolen Street Sign.

It all started one sunny afternoon, as the residents of Quirktown strolled through the town square, admiring the colorful storefronts and quirky decorations. But as they rounded the corner onto Main Street, they were met with a peculiar sight: the street sign for "Main Street" was missing!

The local news ran headlines declaring, "Quirktown's Curious Conundrum: The Case of the Stolen Street Sign Leaves Town in a Tizzy!"

But amidst the confusion and commotion, there were moments of sheer absurdity as the residents of Quirktown attempted to solve the mystery. Some speculated that aliens had abducted the sign, while others pointed fingers at rival towns in a sign-stealing feud.

But the true heroes of the day were a group of elderly ladies known as the "Sign Sleuths," who had unwittingly become the darlings of Quirktown with their amateur detective skills and colorful personalities. With magnifying glasses in hand and determination in their hearts, they set out to crack the case.

From that day forward, Quirktown became known as the town that had a close encounter with the sign-stealing kind, a place where even the most peculiar of mysteries could be solved with a little laughter and a lot of community spirit.

And so, as the residents of Quirktown bid farewell to The Case of the Stolen Street Sign and returned to their daily lives with a smile on their faces and a twinkle in their eyes, they did so knowing that they had been part of a truly whimsical and wonderful adventure.

The Toga Tumult: A Comical Tale of The Great "Toga Party" Escapade

In the lively town of Revelryville, where celebrations were a way of life and laughter filled the air, there occurred an event that would go down in history as The Great "Toga Party" Escapade.

It all began one balmy evening, as the residents of Revelryville gathered for a themed party like no other. The theme? Togas, of course! With bedsheets draped over their shoulders and laurel wreaths adorning their heads, the partygoers were ready to embrace the spirit of ancient Rome.

The local news ran headlines declaring, "Revelryville's Riotous Revels: The Great 'Toga Party' Escapade Leaves Town in Stitches!"

But amidst the merriment and madness, there were moments of sheer hilarity as the residents of Revelryville embraced the toga theme with gusto. Some attempted to speak in faux Latin, while others engaged in spirited debates over who looked the most "Roman."

But the true stars of the show were a group of eccentric characters known as the Toga Titans, who had unwittingly become the life of the party with their outrageous antics and larger-than-life personalities. With each toga-clad twirl and each hearty laugh, they brought joy and laughter to all who crossed their path.

From that day forward, Revelryville became known as the town that had a close encounter of the toga kind, a place where even the most ordinary of parties could turn into a riotous romp through ancient Rome.

And so, as the residents of Revelryville bid farewell to The Great "Toga Party" Escapade and returned to their daily lives with a smile on their faces and a sheet wrapped around their waists, they did so knowing that they had been part of a truly comical and unforgettable adventure.

The Gorilla-Suit Guffaw: A Whimsical Tale of The Missing Gorilla Suit

In the bustling town of Chuckleville, where laughter was the language and silliness was celebrated, there occurred an event that would go down in history as The Case of the Missing Gorilla Suit.

It all started one sunny day, as the residents of Chuckleville prepared for the annual costume parade. Among the costumes and props, there was one notable absence: the beloved gorilla suit, a staple of the parade for as long as anyone could remember.

The local news ran headlines declaring, "Chuckleville's Comical Crisis: The Case of the Missing Gorilla Suit Leaves Town in a Tizzy!"

But amidst the confusion and chaos, there were moments of sheer hilarity as the residents of Chuckleville attempted to solve the mystery. Some speculated that a real gorilla had taken the suit for a joyride, while others imagined a grand conspiracy involving rival parade participants.

But the true heroes of the day were a group of amateur sleuths known as the Chuckleville Detectives, who had unwittingly become the darlings of the town with their bumbling but enthusiastic investigation. Armed with magnifying glasses and absurd theories, they set out to crack the case.

From that day forward, Chuckleville became known as the town that had a close encounter with the gorilla-suit kind, a place where even the most peculiar of mysteries could be solved with a little laughter and a lot of community spirit.

And so, as the residents of Chuckleville bid farewell to The Case of the Missing Gorilla Suit and returned to their daily lives with a smile on their faces and a chuckle in their hearts, they did so knowing that they had been part of a truly whimsical and wonderful adventure.

The Whoopee Cushion Caper: A Hilarious Tale of The Prank Gone Pffft!

In the jolly town of Chuckleville, where laughter was the currency and silliness was celebrated, there occurred an event that would go down in history as The "Whoopee Cushion" Prank.

It all began on a sunny afternoon, as the residents of Chuckleville gathered for a neighborhood barbecue. Among the burgers and hotdogs, there was one item that stood out: a lone whoopee cushion strategically placed on a chair.

The local news ran headlines declaring, "Chuckleville's Chucklefest: The Great 'Whoopee Cushion' Prank Leaves Town in Stitches!"

But amidst the laughter and chaos, there were moments of sheer hilarity as the residents of Chuckleville attempted to solve the mystery of the phantom tooter. Some blamed it on the wind, while others pointed fingers at the neighbor's dog.

But the true prankster of the day was a mischievous youngster named Joey, who had unwittingly become the hero of Chuckleville with his ingenious prank. With a sly grin and a well-placed whoopee cushion, he had the entire town laughing until their sides hurt.

From that day forward, Chuckleville became known as the town that had a close encounter with the whoopee cushion kind, a place where even the most unexpected of pranks could bring people together in laughter and camaraderie.

And so, as the residents of Chuckleville bid farewell to The "Whoopee Cushion" Prank and returned to their daily lives with a smile on their faces and a chuckle in their hearts, they did so knowing that they had been part of a truly pffft-tastic and hilarious adventure.

The Watery Wobble: A Splashy Tale of The Great "Waterbed" Fad

Once upon a time, in the cozy town of Splashville, where laughter flowed like a river and silliness was the norm, there occurred an event that would go down in history as The Great "Waterbed" Fad.

It all started one sunny day, as the residents of Splashville caught wind of the latest craze sweeping the nation: waterbeds. These squishy, wobbly mattresses filled with water promised a night of sleep like no other.

The local news ran headlines declaring, "Splashville's Soggy Sensation: The Great 'Waterbed' Fad Leaves Town in a Wobble!"

But amidst the excitement and laughter, there were moments of sheer hilarity as the residents of Splashville embraced the waterbed trend with gusto. Some attempted to bounce on their beds like oversized water balloons, while others found themselves rolling off the edges in fits of laughter.

But the true stars of the show were a group of adventurous souls known as the Aqua Dreamers, who had unwittingly become the champions of Splashville with their daring dives and epic waterbed battles. With each splash and each wobble, they brought joy and laughter to all who joined in the fun.

From that day forward, Splashville became known as the town that had a close encounter of the watery kind, a place where even the most peculiar of fads could bring people together in laughter and camaraderie.

And so, as the residents of Splashville bid farewell to The Great "Waterbed" Fad and returned to their dry, land-based lives with a smile on their faces and a squish in their step, they did so knowing that they had been part of a truly wobbly and wonderful adventure.

Let's go Back

To the 80's

The Cabbage Caper: A Zany Tale of The Great Cabbage Patch Kids Craze

Once upon a time, in the cozy town of Veggieville, where gardens flourished and laughter sprouted like weeds, there occurred an event that would go down in history as The Great Cabbage Patch Kids Craze.

It all began one sunny day, as the residents of Veggieville stumbled upon a peculiar sight in the local toy store: rows upon rows of chubby-cheeked dolls with cabbage-shaped heads. These were the Cabbage Patch Kids, and they were taking the town by storm.

The local news ran headlines declaring, "Veggieville's Veggie-Venture: The Great Cabbage Patch Kids Craze Leaves Town in a Pickle!"

But amidst the excitement and laughter, there were moments of sheer hilarity as the residents of Veggieville embraced the Cabbage Patch Kids with gusto. Some attempted to adopt as many dolls as they could carry, while others organized cabbage-themed parades in their honor.

But the true stars of the show were a group of imaginative youngsters known as the Cabbage Crusaders, who had unwittingly become the heroes of Veggieville with their creative play and cabbage-inspired adventures. With each cabbage-patch tea party and each make-believe harvest, they brought joy and laughter to all who joined in the fun.

From that day forward, Veggieville became known as the town that had a close encounter with the leafy kind, a place where even the most unexpected of crazes could bring people together in laughter and camaraderie.

And so, as the residents of Veggieville bid farewell to The Great Cabbage Patch Kids Craze and returned to their daily lives with a smile on their faces and cabbage in their hearts, they did so knowing that they had been part of a truly whimsical and wonderful adventure.

The Mullet Mayhem: A Hairy Tale of The Rise of the Mullets

Once upon a time, in the quirky town of Maneville, where hairstyles were as diverse as the colors of the rainbow and laughter filled the air like hairspray mist, there occurred an event that would go down in history as The Rise of the Mullets.

It all started innocently enough, with a few daring individuals deciding to embrace a hairstyle that was both business in the front and party in the back. Yes, you guessed it – the mullet! With its short length in the front and long, flowing locks in the back, the mullet quickly became the talk of the town.

The local news ran headlines declaring, "Maneville's Mullet Madness: The Rise of the Mullets Leaves Town in Stitches!"

But amidst the chuckles and chortles, there were moments of sheer hilarity as the residents of Maneville embraced the mullet trend with gusto. Some sported mullets so extravagant they defied gravity, while others attempted to style their hair into mullets with varying degrees of success.

But the true heroes of the day were a group of mullet enthusiasts known as the Mane Mavericks, who had unwittingly become the leaders of the mullet movement with their bold fashion choices and unapologetic swagger. With each flip of their luscious locks and each twirl of their mustaches, they brought joy and laughter to all who crossed their path.

From that day forward, Maneville became known as the town that had a close encounter with the hairy kind, a place where even the most outrageous of hairstyles could bring people together in laughter and camaraderie.

And so, as the residents of Maneville bid farewell to The Rise of the Mullets and returned to their daily lives with a smile on their faces and a twinkle in their eyes, they did so knowing that they had been part of a truly follicle-tastic and hilarious adventure.

The Cola Catastrophe: A Fizzy Tale of The Infamous "New Coke" Debacle

Once upon a time, in the bustling town of Sodaville, where soda flowed like a river and bubbles filled the air, there occurred an event that would go down in history as The Infamous "New Coke" Debacle.

It all began with a bold idea from the soda company – they decided to revamp their classic cola recipe and introduce a new and improved version called "New Coke." The news spread like wildfire, and the residents of Sodaville eagerly awaited the arrival of this fizzy newcomer.

The local news ran headlines declaring, "Sodaville's Soda Shake-Up: The Infamous 'New Coke' Debacle Leaves Town in a Fizz!"

But amidst the excitement and anticipation, there were moments of sheer hilarity as the residents of Sodaville tasted the new concoction. Some wrinkled their noses at the unfamiliar flavor, while others attempted to disguise their disappointment with forced smiles.

But the true heroes of the day were a group of soda aficionados known as the Pop Patrol, who had unwittingly become the taste testers of Sodaville with their honest opinions and discerning palates. With each sip and each grimace, they brought laughter and amusement to all who witnessed their reactions.

From that day forward, Sodaville became known as the town that had a close encounter of the carbonated kind, a place where even the most well-intentioned of beverage innovations could go awry.

And so, as the residents of Sodaville bid farewell to The Infamous "New Coke" Debacle and returned to their trusty old cola brands with a smile on their faces and a burp in their bellies, they did so knowing that they had been part of a truly fizzy and funny adventure.

The Pac-Man Pandemonium: A Retro Tale of the "Pac-Man Fever" Phenomenon

Once upon a time, in the pixelated world of Arcadetown, where joysticks clicked and quarters jingled, there occurred an event that would go down in history as The "Pac-Man Fever" Phenomenon.

It all started in the dimly lit arcades, where a new game had taken the town by storm – Pac-Man! With its colorful characters and addictive gameplay, Pac-Man quickly became the talk of the town.

The local news ran headlines declaring, "Arcadetown's Arcade Craze: The 'Pac-Man Fever' Phenomenon Leaves Town in a Maze!"

But amidst the beeps and boops of the arcade machines, there were moments of sheer hilarity as the residents of Arcadetown embraced the Pac-Man craze with gusto. Some spent hours mastering the intricate mazes, while others attempted to mimic the iconic "waka waka" sound effects with varying degrees of success.

But the true heroes of the day were a group of joystick jockeys known as the Pac-Maniacs, who had unwittingly become the champions of Arcadetown with their high scores and lightning-fast reflexes. With each ghostly encounter and each fruit-filled level, they brought joy and laughter to all who watched their gameplay.

From that day forward, Arcadetown became known as the town that had a close encounter with the pixelated kind, a place where even the simplest of games could bring people together in laughter and camaraderie.

And so, as the residents of Arcadetown bid farewell to The "Pac-Man Fever" Phenomenon and returned to their daily lives with a smile on their faces and a pocket full of quarters, they did so knowing that they had been part of a truly retro and hilarious adventure.

The Fashion Fiasco: A Hilarious Tale of Outrageous Fashion Trends

In the bustling town of Styleville, where the sidewalks were runways and the air was filled with the scent of hairspray, there occurred an event that would go down in history as The Outrageous Fashion Trends.

It all started with a few bold individuals deciding to push the boundaries of fashion to new heights, or rather, depths! Suddenly, the streets were filled with people sporting the most outlandish and absurd outfits imaginable.

The local news ran headlines declaring, "Styleville's Stylish Shenanigans: Outrageous Fashion Trends Leave Town in Stitches!"

But amidst the laughter and disbelief, there were moments of sheer hilarity as the residents of Styleville embraced the outrageous fashion trends with gusto. Some strutted down the streets wearing clothing that resembled works of abstract art, while others donned accessories so large they could double as furniture.

But the true stars of the show were a group of fashionistas known as the Trendsetters, who had unwittingly become the darlings of Styleville with their fearless experimentation and avant-garde ensembles. With each daring fashion statement and each exaggerated strut, they brought joy and laughter to all who witnessed their runway-worthy antics.

From that day forward, Styleville became known as the town that had a close encounter of the fashionable kind, a place where even the most outrageous of trends could bring people together in laughter and camaraderie.

And so, as the residents of Styleville bid farewell to The Outrageous Fashion Trends and returned to their more sensible wardrobe choices with a smile on their faces and a chuckle in their hearts, they did so knowing that they had been part of a truly stylish and hilarious adventure.

The Cube Craze: A Whimsical Tale of Rubik's Cube Mania

Once upon a time, in the colorful town of Puzzleville, where logic reigned supreme and creativity flourished, there occurred an event that would go down in history as The Rubik's Cube Mania.

It all started with the arrival of a small, cube-shaped puzzle known as the Rubik's Cube. With its rainbow of colors and perplexing twists and turns, the Rubik's Cube quickly captured the imagination of the townsfolk.

The local news ran headlines declaring, "Puzzleville's Puzzling Pandemonium: Rubik's Cube Mania Leaves Town in a Twist!"

But amidst the confusion and frustration, there were moments of sheer hilarity as the residents of Puzzleville attempted to solve the enigmatic puzzle. Some twisted the cube with determination, while others shook it in hopes of finding a solution.

But the true heroes of the day were a group of puzzle enthusiasts known as the Cube Crusaders, who had unwittingly become the champions of Puzzleville with their unwavering dedication and innovative solving techniques. With each twist and turn of the Rubik's Cube, they brought joy and laughter to all who watched their puzzling prowess.

From that day forward, Puzzleville became known as the town that had a close encounter of the cubical kind, a place where even the most confounding of puzzles could bring people together in laughter and camaraderie.

And so, as the residents of Puzzleville bid farewell to The Rubik's Cube Mania and returned to their daily lives with a smile on their faces and a cube-shaped twinkle in their eyes, they did so knowing that they had been part of a truly puzzling and hilarious adventure.

The Walkman Whimsy: A Comical Tale of the Sony Walkman Introduction

Once upon a time, in the bustling town of Tuneville, where music floated through the air like a catchy melody and laughter danced along the streets, there occurred an event that would go down in history as The Introduction of the Sony Walkman.

It all started with a revolutionary idea from the folks at Sony – a portable music player that could fit in your pocket! The news spread like wildfire, and the residents of Tuneville eagerly awaited the arrival of this new musical marvel.

The local news ran headlines declaring, "Tuneville's Tunesational Transformation: The Introduction of the Sony Walkman Leaves Town in a Musical Frenzy!"

But amidst the excitement and anticipation, there were moments of sheer hilarity as the residents of Tuneville embraced the Walkman with gusto. Some attempted to dance down the streets with their Walkman in hand, while others got tangled in their headphone cords and ended up doing the "Walkman Waltz" instead.

But the true heroes of the day were a group of music lovers known as the Tune Titans, who had unwittingly become the ambassadors of Tuneville's musical revolution with their eclectic playlists and spontaneous dance parties. With each catchy beat and each off-key sing-along, they brought joy and laughter to all who joined in the musical mayhem.

From that day forward, Tuneville became known as the town that had a close encounter of the musical kind, a place where even the simplest of inventions could bring people together in laughter and camaraderie.

And so, as the residents of Tuneville bid farewell to The Introduction of the Sony Walkman and returned to their daily lives with a smile on their faces and a song in their hearts, they did so knowing that they had been part of a truly tuneful and hilarious adventure.

The Aerobics Antics: A Laugh-Out-Loud Tale of Hilarious Workout Videos

Once upon a time, in the lively town of Fitville, where exercise was celebrated and laughter echoed through the gym halls, there occurred an event that would go down in history as The Hilarious Aerobics Workout Videos.

It all started with a burst of energy from fitness enthusiasts who decided to share their workout routines on video. The news spread like wildfire, and the residents of Fitville eagerly awaited the arrival of these new exercise guides.

The local news ran headlines declaring, "Fitville's Fitness Frenzy: The Hilarious Aerobics Workout Videos Leave Town in Stitches!"

But amidst the sweat and silliness, there were moments of sheer hilarity as the residents of Fitville followed along with the workout videos. Some attempted to mimic the instructors' moves with precision, while others stumbled and tripped over their own feet in fits of laughter.

But the true heroes of the day were a group of workout warriors known as the Sweat Squad, who had unwittingly become the stars of Fitville's fitness craze with their enthusiastic participation and unforgettable dance moves. With each grapevine step and each jazz hand flourish, they brought joy and laughter to all who joined in the aerobic antics.

From that day forward, Fitville became known as the town that had a close encounter of the aerobic kind, a place where even the most challenging of workouts could bring people together in laughter and camaraderie.

And so, as the residents of Fitville bid farewell to The Hilarious Aerobics Workout Videos and returned to their daily lives with a smile on their faces and a spring in their step, they did so knowing that they had been part of a truly hilarious and heart-pumping adventure.

The Hair-Raising Hilarity: A Rockin' Tale of Hair Metal Bands

Once upon a time, in the electrifying town of Rockville, where guitars wailed and drums pounded like thunder, there occurred an event that would go down in history as The Absurdity of Hair Metal Bands.

It all started with a group of musicians who decided to take the rock 'n' roll scene by storm with their flamboyant style and gravity-defying hairstyles. The news spread like wildfire, and the residents of Rockville eagerly awaited the arrival of these new musical marvels.

The local news ran headlines declaring, "Rockville's Rock 'n' Roll Revolution: The Absurdity of Hair Metal Bands Leaves Town in a Mullet-Fueled Frenzy!"

But amidst the hair spray and leather pants, there were moments of sheer hilarity as the residents of Rockville witnessed the spectacle of hair metal bands in action. Some marveled at the musicians' outrageous outfits and teased hair, while others couldn't help but chuckle at the over-the-top theatrics.

But the true heroes of the day were a group of rock enthusiasts known as the Head Bangers, who had unwittingly become the champions of Rockville's hair metal scene with their wild air guitar solos and enthusiastic head-banging. With each power chord and each high-pitched scream, they brought joy and laughter to all who rocked out with them.

From that day forward, Rockville became known as the town that had a close encounter of the hair-raising kind, a place where even the most absurd of musical trends could bring people together in laughter and camaraderie.

And so, as the residents of Rockville bid farewell to The Absurdity of Hair Metal Bands and returned to their daily lives with a smile on their faces and a riff in their hearts, they did so knowing that they had been part of a truly rockin' and hilarious adventure.

The Silly Sayings Saga: A Chuckle-Worthy Tale of The "Just Say No" Campaign

Once upon a time, in the quirky town of Wordville, where words were the currency and laughter filled the air like punctuation marks, there occurred an event that would go down in history as The "Just Say No" Campaign.

It all started with a well-intentioned initiative to discourage people from using drugs by promoting the catchy slogan "Just Say No." The news spread like a misplaced comma, and the residents of Wordville eagerly awaited the impact of this new campaign.

The local news ran headlines declaring, "Wordville's Wacky Wordsmiths: The 'Just Say No' Campaign Leaves Town in a Tongue-Tied Tizzy!"

But amidst the serious message, there were moments of sheer hilarity as the residents of Wordville attempted to incorporate the slogan into their daily conversations. Some replied with "Just say no" to offers of dessert, while others found themselves awkwardly blurting out the phrase at the most unexpected moments.

But the true heroes of the day were a group of language enthusiasts known as the Tongue Twisters, who had unwittingly become the champions of Wordville's linguistic chaos with their creative interpretations of the slogan. With each tongue-tied attempt and each misplaced "no," they brought joy and laughter to all who listened.

From that day forward, Wordville became known as the town that had a close encounter of the silly saying kind, a place where even the most serious of campaigns could bring people together in laughter and camaraderie.

And so, as the residents of Wordville bid farewell to The "Just Say No" Campaign and returned to their daily lives with a smile on their faces and a pun in their hearts, they did so knowing that they had been part of a truly chuckle-worthy and memorable adventure.

The Zany Zeal of "Weird Al": A Whimsical Tale of Popularity

Once upon a time, in the uproarious town of Quirkville, where laughter echoed through the streets and creativity flourished like dandelions in spring, there occurred an event that would go down in history as The Popularity of "Weird Al" Yankovic.

It all started with a man named Al, whose peculiar talent for parodying popular songs captured the hearts of the townsfolk. The news spread faster than a runaway pun, and the residents of Quirkville eagerly awaited each new musical creation from the zany entertainer.

The local news ran headlines declaring, "Quirkville's Musical Mirth: The Popularity of 'Weird Al' Yankovic Leaves Town in Stitches!"

But amidst the laughter and delight, there were moments of sheer hilarity as the residents of Quirkville listened to "Weird Al's" offbeat renditions of their favorite tunes. Some found themselves singing along with his quirky lyrics, while others couldn't help but chuckle at his humorous music videos.

But the true heroes of the day were a group of "Weird Al" enthusiasts known as the Quirky Crew, who had unwittingly become the champions of Quirkville's musical scene with their undying devotion to the parody master. With each accordion riff and each comical verse, they brought joy and laughter to all who tuned in to "Weird Al's" antics.

From that day forward, Quirkville became known as the town that had a close encounter of the zany kind, a place where even the most unusual of entertainers could bring people together in laughter and camaraderie.

And so, as the residents of Quirkville bid farewell to The Popularity of "Weird Al" Yankovic and continued to sing his silly songs with a smile on their faces and a skip in their steps, they did so knowing that they had been part of a truly whimsical and entertaining adventure.

The Groovy Ghoul Gala: A Spooky Tale of The Thriller Dance Craze

Once upon a time, in the spirited town of Spooksville, where ghosts roamed freely and skeletons danced in the moonlight, there occurred an event that would go down in history as The Thriller Dance Craze.

It all started with a hauntingly catchy tune and a mesmerizing dance routine from the King of Pop, Michael Jackson. The news spread like wildfire, and the residents of Spooksville eagerly awaited their chance to join in on the spine-tingling fun.

The local news ran headlines declaring, "Spooksville's Spectacular Specter Shindig: The Thriller Dance Craze Leaves Town in a Frightful Frenzy!"

But amidst the eerie atmosphere, there were moments of sheer hilarity as the residents of Spooksville attempted to master the iconic Thriller dance moves. Some twisted and twirled with frightening precision, while others stumbled and comically tripped over their own feet.

But the true stars of the show were a group of undead enthusiasts known as the Ghoulish Gang, who had unwittingly become the champions of Spooksville's dance craze with their spirited performances and bone-rattling enthusiasm. With each moonwalk and each zombie shuffle, they brought joy and laughter to all who joined in the spooky spectacle.

From that day forward, Spooksville became known as the town that had a close encounter of the eerie kind, a place where even the most chilling of dances could bring people together in laughter and camaraderie.

And so, as the residents of Spooksville bid farewell to The Thriller Dance Craze and continued to bust out their best moves with a smile on their faces and a shimmy in their step, they did so knowing that they had been part of a truly groovy and hilarious adventure.

The Punk Rock Pandemonium: A Riotous Tale of Rebellion

Once upon a time, in the rebellious town of Riotville, where chaos reigned and anarchy was the order of the day, there occurred an event that would go down in history as The Rise of Punk Rock.

It all started with a few disenchanted youths who decided to pick up guitars, bang on drums, and scream into microphones to express their frustration with the status quo. The news spread like wildfire, and the residents of Riotville eagerly awaited the arrival of this new musical revolution.

The local news ran headlines declaring, "Riotville's Rambunctious Revolution: The Rise of Punk Rock Leaves Town in a Mosh Pit Mayhem!"

But amidst the chaos and cacophony, there were moments of sheer hilarity as the residents of Riotville embraced the punk rock movement with gusto. Some dyed their hair outrageous colors and pierced their bodies with safety pins, while others attempted to slam dance with the grace of a newborn giraffe.

But the true heroes of the day were a group of punk enthusiasts known as the Rebel Rousers, who had unwittingly become the champions of Riotville's musical uprising with their DIY ethos and devil-may-care attitude. With each raucous chord and each defiant shout, they brought joy and laughter to all who joined in the punk rock pandemonium.

From that day forward, Riotville became known as the town that had a close encounter of the rebellious kind, a place where even the most unconventional of music genres could bring people together in laughter and camaraderie.

And so, as the residents of Riotville bid farewell to The Rise of Punk Rock and continued to rock out with a smile on their faces and a safety pin in their ears, they did so knowing that they had been part of a truly riotous and hilarious adventure.

The Silly Saturday Shenanigans: A Whimsical Tale of Saturday Morning Cartoons

Once upon a time, in the zany world of Cartoonville, where colors were brighter than a rainbow and laughter echoed through the streets like a catchy tune, there occurred an event that would go down in history as The Wacky World of Saturday Morning Cartoons.

It all started when the sun peeked over the horizon, and children across the land jumped out of bed with glee, knowing that it was Saturday – the day when their favorite cartoons graced the television screen. The news spread like confetti, and the residents of Cartoonville eagerly awaited the antics of their beloved animated characters.

The local news ran headlines declaring, "Cartoonville's Comical Craze: The Wacky World of Saturday Morning Cartoons Leaves Town in Stitches!"

But amidst the laughter and excitement, there were moments of sheer hilarity as the residents of Cartoonville tuned in to their favorite shows. Some giggled at the misadventures of wacky animals, while others marveled at the absurdity of superheroes with super-sized egos.

But the true heroes of the day were a group of cartoon connoisseurs known as the Toon Team, who had unwittingly become the champions of Cartoonville's animated realm with their encyclopedic knowledge of characters and catchphrases. With each slapstick gag and each witty one-liner, they brought joy and laughter to all who joined in the Saturday morning cartoon extravaganza.

From that day forward, Cartoonville became known as the town that had a close encounter of the animated kind, a place where even the most fantastical of worlds could bring people together in laughter and camaraderie.

And so, as the residents of Cartoonville bid farewell to The Wacky World of Saturday Morning Cartoons and continued to laugh along with their favorite characters with a smile on their faces and a bowl of cereal in their hands, they did so knowing that they had been part of a truly hilarious and unforgettable adventure.

The Dismal Delorean Disaster: A Hilarious Tale of Epic Fail

Once upon a time, in the bustling town of Motorville, where cars ruled the roads and engines roared like lions, there occurred an event that would go down in history as The Epic Fail of the DeLorean DMC-12.

It all started with a sleek and futuristic car known as the DeLorean DMC-12, touted as the vehicle of the future with its gull-wing doors and stainless-steel exterior. The news spread like a flat tire, and the residents of Motorville eagerly awaited their chance to drive this automotive marvel.

The local news ran headlines declaring, "Motorville's Mishap Madness: The Epic Fail of the DeLorean DMC-12 Leaves Town in a Fender-Bender Frenzy!"

But amidst the excitement and anticipation, there were moments of sheer hilarity as the residents of Motorville experienced the pitfalls of the DeLorean DMC-12. Some struggled to open the stubborn gull-wing doors, while others found themselves stuck in traffic as the car sputtered and stalled.

But the true heroes of the day were a group of car enthusiasts known as the Road Warriors, who had unwittingly become the champions of Motorville's automotive mishaps with their humorous anecdotes and roadside rescues. With each breakdown and each roadside repair, they brought joy and laughter to all who encountered the DMC-12's epic fail.

From that day forward, Motorville became known as the town that had a close encounter of the car-related kind, a place where even the most hyped-up vehicles could bring people together in laughter and camaraderie.

And so, as the residents of Motorville bid farewell to The Epic Fail of the DeLorean DMC-12 and continued to cruise the streets with a smile on their faces and a spare tire in their trunk, they did so knowing that they had been part of a truly hilarious and unforgettable automotive adventure.

The VHS Vendetta: A Hilarious Tale of Video Rental Store Invasion

Once upon a time, in the cozy town of Movieville, where film reels spun and popcorn popped like fireworks, there occurred an event that would go down in history as The Invasion of Video Rental Stores.

It all started with the arrival of video rental stores, promising endless entertainment at the touch of a button. The news spread like spilled soda, and the residents of Movieville eagerly awaited their chance to peruse the aisles of cinematic treasures.

The local news ran headlines declaring, "Movieville's Movie Madness: The Invasion of Video Rental Stores Leaves Town in a Reel Frenzy!"

But amidst the excitement and anticipation, there were moments of sheer hilarity as the residents of Movieville navigated the labyrinthine aisles of the video rental stores. Some wandered, overwhelmed by the sheer number of movie options, while others got tangled in the endless rows of VHS tapes like hapless heroes in a movie marathon gone wrong.

But the true heroes of the day were a group of film buffs known as the Movie Mavericks, who had unwittingly become the champions of Movieville's cinematic chaos with their humorous reviews and movie night mishaps. With each cheesy movie selection and each late fee incurred, they brought joy and laughter to all who ventured into the world of video rentals.

From that day forward, Movieville became known as the town that had a close encounter of the cinematic kind, a place where even the most outrageous of movie plots could bring people together in laughter and camaraderie.

And so, as the residents of Movieville bid farewell to The Invasion of Video Rental Stores and continued to enjoy movie nights with a smile on their faces and a bucket of popcorn in their laps, they did so knowing that they had been part of a truly hilarious and unforgettable film frenzy.

The Beefy Blunder: A Chuckle-Inducing Tale of the "Where's the Beef?" Catchphrase

Once upon a time, in the bustling town of Hungryville, where stomachs growled and cravings roamed free, there occurred an event that would go down in history as "Where's the Beef?" Catchphrase.

It all started with a catchy commercial for a fast-food chain featuring three elderly ladies inspecting a hamburger bun, one of whom famously exclaimed, "Where's the beef?" The news spread like melted cheese on a burger, and the residents of Hungryville eagerly awaited their chance to use the now-iconic catchphrase.

The local news ran headlines declaring, "Hungryville's Hilarious Hamburger Hubbub: The 'Where's the Beef?' Catchphrase Leaves Town in a Patty Patty Frenzy!"

But amidst the hunger and anticipation, there were moments of sheer hilarity as the residents of Hungryville incorporated the catchphrase into their daily conversations. Some asked for extra toppings on their burgers, only to quip, "Where's the beef?" while others playfully used the phrase to express their disappointment in anything lacking substance.

But the true heroes of the day were a group of foodies known as the Burger Brigade, who had unwittingly become the champions of Hungryville's culinary comedy with their creative use of the catchphrase. With each beefy joke and each cheesy pun, they brought joy and laughter to all who indulged in the deliciously funny atmosphere.

From that day forward, Hungryville became known as the town that had a close encounter of the beefy kind, a place where even the simplest of catchphrases could bring people together in laughter and camaraderie.

And so, as the residents of Hungryville bid farewell to The "Where's the Beef?" Catchphrase and continued to enjoy their favorite meals with a smile on their faces and a hearty appetite in their hearts, they did so knowing that they had been part of a truly hilarious and mouthwatering adventure.

The Hair-Raising Harmonies: A Hilarious Tale of Hair Bands' Ballads

Once upon a time, in the lively town of Rockville, where guitars wailed and drums thundered like a storm, there occurred an event that would go down in history as The Absurdity of Hair Bands' Ballads.

It all started with the rise of hair bands, whose members boasted towering hairstyles and an affinity for heartfelt ballads. The news spread like wildfire, and the residents of Rockville eagerly awaited their chance to rock out to these melodramatic tunes.

The local news ran headlines declaring, "Rockville's Riotous Rock Ballad Revival: The Absurdity of Hair Bands' Ballads Leaves Town in Tears of Laughter!"

But amidst the hairspray and spandex, there were moments of sheer hilarity as the residents of Rockville listened to the over-the-top ballads of the hair bands. Some couldn't help but chuckle at the overly dramatic lyrics about heartbreak and longing, while others found themselves rolling their eyes at the extravagant music videos featuring wind machines and flying hair.

But the true heroes of the day were a group of music lovers known as the Rock Rebels, who had unwittingly become the champions of Rockville's rock ballad ridicule with their humorous commentary and air guitar solos. With each exaggerated wail and each melodramatic chord progression, they brought joy and laughter to all who rocked out with them.

From that day forward, Rockville became known as the town that had a close encounter of the absurdly emotional kind, a place where even the most theatrical of rock ballads could bring people together in laughter and camaraderie.

And so, as the residents of Rockville bid farewell to The Absurdity of Hair Bands' Ballads and continued to enjoy their favorite tunes with a smile on their faces and headbangs in their hearts, they did so knowing that they had been part of a truly hilarious and unforgettable musical adventure.

The Comical Conundrum of Early Computers: A Laughable Tale of Technological Awkwardness

Once upon a time, in the quaint town of Byteville, where wires tangled and screens flickered like fireflies, there occurred an event that would go down in history as The Awkwardness of Early Computer Technology.

It all started with the arrival of early computers, clunky machines that whirred and beeped with all the grace of a clumsy robot. The news spread like a computer virus, and the residents of Byteville eagerly awaited their chance to dive into the world of digital wonders.

The local news ran headlines declaring, "Byteville's Bumbling Bits and Bytes: The Awkwardness of Early Computer Technology Leaves Town in a Tangled Web!"

But amidst the excitement and anticipation, there were moments of sheer hilarity as the residents of Byteville grappled with the quirks of early computer technology. Some struggled to understand the concept of floppy disks, while others found themselves lost in a maze of DOS commands and error messages.

But the true heroes of the day were a group of tech enthusiasts known as the Geek Squad, who had unwittingly become the champions of Byteville's technological turmoil with their humorous troubleshooting and endless patience. With each crashed program and each frozen screen, they brought joy and laughter to all who encountered the awkwardness of early computers.

From that day forward, Byteville became known as the town that had a close encounter of the digital kind, a place where even the most awkward of technological advances could bring people together in laughter and camaraderie.

And so, as the residents of Byteville bid farewell to The Awkwardness of Early Computer Technology and continued to embrace the digital age with a smile on their faces and a mouse in their hands, they did so knowing that they had been part of a truly hilarious and unforgettable technological adventure.

The Miami Vice Fashion Fiasco: A Riotous Tale of Outrageousness

Once upon a time, in the vibrant city of Miami, where palm trees swayed and neon lights flashed like disco balls, there occurred an event that would go down in history as The Outrageousness of "Miami Vice" Fashion.

It all started with the iconic TV show "Miami Vice," which brought the city's vibrant culture to screens across the nation. The news spread like wildfire, and fashionistas everywhere eagerly awaited their chance to emulate the show's signature style.

The local news ran headlines declaring, "Miami's Magnificent Mayhem: The Outrageousness of 'Miami Vice' Fashion Leaves Town in a Neon Glow!"

But amidst the excitement and anticipation, there were moments of sheer hilarity as people attempted to replicate the show's fashion choices. Some sported pastel-colored suits and loafers without socks, while others donned oversized sunglasses and flashy jewelry in an attempt to capture the show's Miami chic.

But the true heroes of the day were a group of trendsetters known as the Vice Squad, who had unwittingly become the champions of Miami's fashion frenzy with their bold choices and unapologetic embrace of all things "Miami Vice." With each rolled-up sleeve and each popped collar, they brought joy and laughter to all who dared to join in the outrageousness of "Miami Vice" fashion.

From that day forward, Miami became known as the city that had a close encounter of the stylish kind, a place where even the most outlandish of fashion trends could bring people together in laughter and camaraderie.

And so, as the residents of Miami bid farewell to The Outrageousness of "Miami Vice" Fashion and continued to strut their stuff with a smile on their faces and a flair for the dramatic, they did so knowing that they had been part of a truly hilarious and unforgettable fashion adventure.

Let's go Back
To the 90's

The Beanie Baby Bonanza: A Whimsical Tale of Furry Frenzy

Once upon a time, in the cozy town of Beanieville, where stitches were stitched and fluff fluffed like a magical spell, there occurred an event that would go down in history as The Beanie Baby Craze.

It all started with the arrival of Beanie Babies, tiny plush toys filled with beans that captured the hearts of collectors far and wide. The news spread like a wave of cuddly cuteness, and the residents of Beanieville eagerly awaited their chance to add these adorable critters to their collections.

The local news ran headlines declaring, "Beanieville's Bursting Beanie Bubble: The Beanie Baby Craze Leaves Town in a Flurry of Fur!"

But amidst the excitement and anticipation, there were moments of sheer hilarity as the residents of Beanieville scrambled to collect as many Beanie Babies as possible. Some lined up outside toy stores for hours, while others traded Beanie Babies like rare treasures in a quest to complete their collections.

But the true heroes of the day were a group of collectors known as the Beanie Brigade, who had unwittingly become the champions of Beanieville's furry frenzy with their dedication and enthusiasm. With each new addition to their collections and each Beanie Baby trade, they brought joy and laughter to all who joined in the Beanie Baby bonanza.

From that day forward, Beanieville became known as the town that had a close encounter of the plush kind, a place where even the smallest of toys could bring people together in laughter and camaraderie.

And so, as the residents of Beanieville bid farewell to The Beanie Baby Craze and continued to cherish their collections with a smile on their faces and a Beanie Baby in their hands, they did so knowing that they had been part of a truly hilarious and heartwarming plush toy adventure.

The Macarena Mayhem: A Hilarious Tale of Dancefloor Delirium

Once upon a time, in the lively town of Groovetown, where beats boomed and hips swayed like palm trees in a breeze, there occurred an event that would go down in history as The Macarena Madness.

It all started with a catchy Spanish song called "Macarena," with a dance routine so infectious it swept the nation faster than a tidal wave of rhythm. The news spread like wildfire, and the residents of Groovetown eagerly awaited their chance to bust out the iconic moves.

The local news ran headlines declaring, "Groovetown's Groovy Galore: The Macarena Madness Leaves Town in a Dancefloor Daze!"

But amidst the excitement and anticipation, there were moments of sheer hilarity as the residents of Groovetown attempted to master the

Macarena dance. Some flailed their arms like windmills, while others stumbled over their own feet in a comical attempt to keep up with the rhythm.

But the true heroes of the day were a group of dance enthusiasts known as the Macarena Maniacs, who had unwittingly become the champions of Groovetown's dancefloor delirium with their spirited performances and infectious enthusiasm. With each twist and each turn, they brought joy and laughter to all who joined in the Macarena madness.

From that day forward, Groovetown became known as the town that had a close encounter of the groovy kind, a place where even the simplest of dance moves could bring people together in laughter and camaraderie.

And so, as the residents of Groovetown bid farewell to The Macarena Madness and continued to boogie on with a smile on their faces and a shimmy in their steps, they did so knowing that they had been part of a truly hilarious and unforgettable dancefloor adventure.

The Tamagotchi Tumult: A Comical Tale of Digital Pet Pandemonium

Once upon a time, in the bustling town of Gizmoville, where gadgets beeped and screens blinked like fireflies, there occurred an event that would go down in history as The Introduction of Tamagotchis.

It all started with the arrival of Tamagotchis, tiny digital pets housed in egg-shaped devices that captured the hearts of children and adults alike. The news spread like wildfire, and the residents of Gizmoville eagerly awaited their chance to care for these virtual critters.

The local news ran headlines declaring, "Gizmoville's Gigantic Gizmo Gala: The Introduction of Tamagotchis Leaves Town in a Digital Daze!"

But amidst the excitement and anticipation, there were moments of sheer hilarity as the residents of Gizmoville struggled to keep their Tamagotchis alive. Some fed their digital pets incessantly, while others forgot to clean up their virtual messes in a comedic frenzy of forgetfulness.

But the true heroes of the day were a group of Tamagotchi aficionados known as the Pixel Pets, who had unwittingly become the champions of Gizmoville's digital pet pandemonium with their dedication and determination. With each pixelated chirp and each virtual wag of the tail, they brought joy and laughter to all who joined in the Tamagotchi tumult.

From that day forward, Gizmoville became known as the town that had a close encounter of the digital kind, a place where even the tiniest of gadgets could bring people together in laughter and camaraderie.

And so, as the residents of Gizmoville bid farewell to The Introduction of Tamagotchis and continued to care for their virtual pets with a smile on their faces and a button press in their hands, they did so knowing that they had been part of a truly hilarious and unforgettable digital adventure.

The Boy Band Boom: A Cheeky Tale of Crooning Charm

Once upon a time, in the melodious town of Harmonyville, where harmonies harmonized and hearts swooned like lovesick kittens, there occurred an event that would go down in history as The Surge of Boy Bands.

It all started with the rise of boy bands, groups of charming young lads crooning their way into the hearts of fans around the world. The news spread like a catchy chorus, and the residents of Harmonyville eagerly awaited their chance to swoon over these musical heartthrobs.

The local news ran headlines declaring, "Harmonyville's Harmonious Hullabaloo: The Surge of Boy Bands Leaves Town in a Melodic Muddle!"

But amidst the excitement and anticipation, there were moments of sheer hilarity as the residents of Harmonyville embraced the boy band craze. Some screamed their lungs out at concerts, while others adorned their walls with posters of their favorite band members in a frenzy of fanatical fervor.

But the true heroes of the day were a group of boy band aficionados known as the Harmony Hysterics, who had unwittingly become the champions of Harmonyville's crooning charm with their dedication and enthusiasm. With each swoon and each serenade, they brought joy and laughter to all who joined in the boy band boom.

From that day forward, Harmonyville became known as the town that had a close encounter of the melodic kind, a place where even the cheesiest of pop tunes could bring people together in laughter and camaraderie.

And so, as the residents of Harmonyville bid farewell to The Surge of Boy Bands and continued to sing along with a smile on their faces and a beat in their hearts, they did so knowing that they had been part of a truly hilarious and unforgettable musical adventure.

The Fresh Prince Fiasco: A Zany Tale of Sitcom Shenanigans

Once upon a time, in the sunny city of Bel-Air, where mansions gleamed and palm trees swayed like hip-hop dancers, there occurred an event that would go down in history as The Hilarity of "The Fresh Prince of Bel-Air".

It all started with a TV show called "The Fresh Prince of Bel-Air," featuring a young rapper named Will Smith who moves from the mean streets of Philadelphia to live with his wealthy relatives in California. The news spread like a catchy rap, and viewers everywhere eagerly awaited their chance to tune in to the comedic chaos.

The local news ran headlines declaring, "Bel-Air's Bellyaching Bonanza: The Hilarity of 'The Fresh Prince of Bel-Air' Leaves Town in Stitches!"

But amidst the laughter and anticipation, there were moments of sheer hilarity as viewers watched Will Smith navigate the ups and downs of life in Bel-Air. Some chuckled at his fish-out-of-water antics, while others marveled at the witty banter and catchy theme song in a riotous wave of sitcom silliness.

But the true heroes of the day were a group of sitcom enthusiasts known as the Bel-Air Buffoons, who had unwittingly become the champions of Bel-Air's sitcom shenanigans with their humorous commentary and infectious laughter. With each punchline and each pratfall, they brought joy and laughter to all who tuned in to "The Fresh Prince of Bel-Air".

From that day forward, Bel-Air became known as the city that had a close encounter of the sitcom kind, a place where even the most outrageous of sitcoms could bring people together in laughter and camaraderie.

And so, as the residents of Bel-Air bid farewell to The Hilarity of "The Fresh Prince of Bel-Air" and continued to reminisce about their favorite episodes with a smile on their faces and a chuckle in their hearts, they did so knowing that they had been part of a truly hilarious and unforgettable sitcom adventure.

The Pokémon Pandemonium: A Wacky Tale of Pocket Monsters

Once upon a time, in the bustling town of Pokéville, where creatures roamed and trainers trained like champions, there occurred an event that would go down in history as Pokémon Mania.

It all started with the release of Pokémon, a video game and trading card phenomenon that captured the imaginations of kids and adults alike. The news spread like wildfire, and the residents of Pokéville eagerly awaited their chance to catch 'em all.

The local news ran headlines declaring, "Pokéville's Perplexing Pokémon Parade: The Pokémon Mania Leaves Town in a Pokéball Frenzy!"

But amidst the excitement and anticipation, there were moments of sheer hilarity as the residents of Pokéville embarked on their Pokémon adventures. Some wandered the streets with their eyes glued to their Game Boys, while others engaged in epic battles of trading cards in a frenzy of competitive spirit.

But the true heroes of the day were a group of Pokémon enthusiasts known as the Poké Masters, who had unwittingly become the champions of Pokéville's pocket monster pandemonium with their dedication and enthusiasm. With each Pokémon catch and each gym badge earned, they brought joy and laughter to all who joined in the Pokémon craze.

From that day forward, Pokéville became known as the town that had a close encounter with the Pokémon kind, a place where even the most outrageous of creatures could bring people together in laughter and camaraderie.

And so, as the residents of Pokéville bid farewell to The Pokémon Mania and continued to embark on their Pokémon journeys with a smile on their faces and Pokéball in their hands, they did so knowing that they had been part of a truly hilarious and unforgettable Pokémon adventure.

The Cyber Cafe Craze: A Hilarious Tale of Online Odyssey

Once upon a time, in the buzzing town of Netville, where keyboards clacked and screens glowed like neon signs, there occurred an event that would go down in history as The Rise of Internet Cafes.

It all started with the emergence of Internet cafes, cozy spaces where people could surf the web, chat with friends, and sip on cups of java simultaneously. The news spread like a viral meme, and the residents of Netville eagerly awaited their chance to log on to the digital world.

The local news ran headlines declaring, "Netville's Nifty Nook Nirvana: The Rise of Internet Cafes Leaves Town in a Cyber Frenzy!"

But amidst the excitement and anticipation, there were moments of sheer hilarity as the residents of Netville navigated the cyber cafe scene. Some struggled to figure out how to use the mouse, while others accidentally clicked on pop-up ads in a comical display of internet ineptitude.

But the true heroes of the day were a group of cyber aficionados known as the Net Navigators, who had unwittingly become the champions of Netville's online odyssey with their tech-savvy skills and endless patience. With each website visit and each email sent, they brought joy and laughter to all who ventured into the digital realm.

From that day forward, Netville became known as the town that had a close encounter with the cyber kind, a place where even the most technologically challenged could join in the fun of the online world.

And so, as the residents of Netville bid farewell to The Rise of Internet Cafes and continued to surf the web with a smile on their faces and a gigabyte in their hearts, they did so knowing that they had been part of a truly hilarious and unforgettable cyber adventure.

The Y2K Yikes: A Laughable Tale of Millennium Mayhem

Once upon a time, in the jittery town of Millenniumville, where clocks ticked and calendars flipped like a countdown to catastrophe, there occurred an event that would go down in history as The "Y2K" Panic.

It all started with the looming arrival of the year 2000, and rumors swirled about the potential chaos that awaited due to a computer bug called the Y2K bug. The news spread like wildfire, and the residents of Millenniumville eagerly awaited their chance to stock up on supplies and brace themselves for the worst.

The local news ran headlines declaring, "Millenniumville's Madcap Millennium Madness: The 'Y2K' Panic Leaves Town in a Frenzy of Fear!"

But amidst the panic and paranoia, there were moments of sheer hilarity as the residents of Millenniumville prepared for the impending apocalypse. Some hoarded cans of beans and bottles of water, while others fashioned makeshift survival shelters in their basements in a comical display of over-preparedness.

But the true heroes of the day were a group of Y2K enthusiasts known as the Bug Busters, who had unwittingly become the champions of Millenniumville's millennium mayhem with their rational thinking and infectious laughter. With each debunked doomsday theory and each eye roll at the hysteria, they brought joy and relief to all who joined in the Y2K panic.

From that day forward, Millenniumville became known as the town that had a close encounter with the bug kind, a place where even the most outlandish of fears could be faced with humor and resilience.

And so, as the residents of Millenniumville bid farewell to The "Y2K" Panic and continued to live their lives with a smile on their faces and a chuckle in their hearts, they did so knowing that they had been part of a truly hilarious and unforgettable millennium adventure.

The Fanny Pack Fiasco: A Ridiculous Tale of Fashion Faux Pas

Once upon a time, in the fashion-forward town of Styleville, where trends strutted and accessories sparkled like disco balls, there occurred an event that would go down in history as The Absurdity of Fanny Packs.

It all started with the rise of fanny packs, those curious contraptions worn around the waist like a fashion statement gone awry. The news spread like a fashion faux pas, and the residents of Styleville found themselves scratching their heads in bewilderment.

The local news ran headlines declaring, "Styleville's Startling Fanny Pack Saga: The Absurdity Leaves Town in Stitches!"

But amidst the confusion and amusement, there were moments of sheer hilarity as the residents of Styleville tried to make sense of the fanny pack phenomenon. Some attempted to wear them with pride, while others couldn't help but burst into laughter at the sight of them in a comical display of disbelief.

But the true heroes of the day were a group of fashion enthusiasts known as the Trend Trackers, who had unwittingly become the champions of Styleville's fashion folly with their witty commentary and good-natured ribbing. With each exaggerated eye roll and each sarcastic quip, they brought joy and laughter to all who witnessed the absurdity of fanny packs.

From that day forward, Styleville became known as the town that had a close encounter of the fashion kind, a place where even the most outrageous of accessories could bring people together in laughter and camaraderie.

And so, as the residents of Styleville bid farewell to The Absurdity of Fanny Packs and continued to embrace new fashion trends with a smile on their faces and a chuckle in their hearts, they did so knowing that they had been part of a truly hilarious and unforgettable fashion adventure.

The Friends Fiasco: A Hilarious Tale of Sitcom Shenanigans

Once upon a time, in the cozy town of Laughterville, where jokes flew and punchlines zinged like arrows in a comedy duel, there occurred an event that would go down in history as The Comedy of "Friends".

It all started with the debut of a TV show called "Friends," featuring six quirky pals navigating the ups and downs of life in New York City. The news spread like wildfire, and viewers everywhere eagerly tuned in to join the laughter-filled escapades.

The local news ran headlines declaring, "Laughterville's Legendary 'Friends' Laughs: The Comedy Leaves Town in Stitches!"

But amidst the chuckles and guffaws, there were moments of sheer hilarity as viewers watched the antics of Ross, Rachel, Chandler, Monica, Joey, and Phoebe unfold. Some couldn't help but snort with laughter at Chandler's sarcastic wit, while others found themselves in fits of giggles at Joey's dim-witted charm in a comical display of sitcom silliness.

But the true heroes of the day were a group of Friends fanatics known as the Laugh Lovers, who had unwittingly become the champions of Laughterville's sitcom shenanigans with their enthusiastic recitations of iconic lines and spot-on impressions. With each "How you doin'?" and each "We were on a break!", they brought joy and laughter to all who joined in the Friends fiasco.

From that day forward, Laughterville became known as the town that had a close encounter of the sitcom kind, a place where even the most absurd of situations could bring people together in laughter and camaraderie.

And so, as the residents of Laughterville bid farewell to The Comedy of "Friends" and continued to rewatch their favorite episodes with a smile on their faces and a chuckle in their hearts, they did so knowing that they had been part of a truly hilarious and unforgettable sitcom adventure.

The Saved by the Bell Shenanigans: A Zany Tale of Teenage Turmoil

Once upon a time, in the quirky town of Bayside, where lockers slammed and school bells rang like an orchestra of chaos, there occurred an event that would go down in history as The Weirdness of "Saved by the Bell".

It all started with a TV show called "Saved by the Bell", featuring a group of high school students navigating the trials and tribulations of adolescence with exaggerated drama and absurd situations. The news spread like a cafeteria food fight, and viewers everywhere eagerly tuned in to witness the comedic calamities.

The local news ran headlines declaring, "Bayside's Bizarre 'Saved by the Bell' Ballyhoo: The Weirdness Leaves Town in Fits of Laughter!"

But amidst the laughter and eye-rolling, there were moments of sheer hilarity as viewers watched Zack, Kelly, Slater, Jessie, Screech, and Lisa stumble their way through high school. Some couldn't help but chuckle at Zack's scheming antics, while others found themselves shaking their heads at Screech's quirky inventions in a comical display of teenage turmoil.

But the true heroes of the day were a group of "Saved by the Bell" enthusiasts known as the Bayside Buffoons, who had unwittingly become the champions of Bayside's sitcom weirdness with their enthusiastic reenactments and inside jokes. With each "Time out!" and each "Preppy!" shout, they brought joy and laughter to all who joined in the Saved by the Bell shenanigans.

From that day forward, Bayside became known as the town that had a close encounter of the sitcom kind, a place where even the most absurd of teenage hijinks could bring people together in laughter and camaraderie.

And so, as the residents of Bayside bid farewell to The Weirdness of "Saved by the Bell" and continued to reminisce about their favorite episodes with a smile on their faces and a shake of their heads, they did so knowing that they had been part of a truly hilarious and unforgettable sitcom adventure.

The Baywatch Brouhaha: A Beachy Tale of Bizarre Lifeguarding

Once upon a time, in the sunny paradise of Baywatch Beach, where waves crashed and sunscreen flowed like coconut-scented dreams, there occurred an event that would go down in history as The Absurdity of "Baywatch".

It all started with a TV show called "Baywatch", featuring a team of lifeguards patrolling the shores of sunny California with impeccable hair and beach-ready bodies. The news spread like a ripple in the ocean, and viewers everywhere eagerly tuned in to witness the melodramatic rescues and beachside antics.

The local news ran headlines declaring, "Baywatch Beach's Bewildering 'Baywatch' Buffoonery: The Absurdity Leaves Town in Sandy Stitches!"

But amidst the slow-motion running and slo-mo hair flips, there were moments of sheer hilarity as viewers watched Mitch, C.J., Hobie, and the rest of the Baywatch crew navigate the highs and lows of beach life. Some couldn't help but laugh at the over-the-top rescues, while others found themselves rolling their eyes at the dramatic dialogue in a comical display of beachside absurdity.

But the true heroes of the day were a group of "Baywatch" enthusiasts known as the Beach Bums, who had unwittingly become the champions of Baywatch Beach's lifeguarding lunacy with their enthusiastic reenactments and beach-themed parties. With each "Hey, Mitch!" and each slow-motion dive, they brought joy and laughter to all who joined in the Baywatch brouhaha.

From that day forward, Baywatch Beach became known as the town that had a close encounter of the beachside kind, a place where even the most absurd of lifeguarding adventures could bring people together in laughter and camaraderie.

And so, as the residents of Baywatch Beach bid farewell to The Absurdity of "Baywatch" and continued to soak up the sun with a smile on their faces and a wink to the lifeguards, they did so knowing that they had been part of a truly hilarious and unforgettable beachside adventure.

The Pog Pandemonium: A Wacky Tale of Slammer Slapstick

Once upon a time, in the bustling town of Pogsville, where cardboard discs flipped and plastic slammers clashed like a chaotic carnival, there occurred an event that would go down in history as The Craziness of Pogs.

It all started with the arrival of Pogs, those curious collectible discs adorned with colorful designs and quirky characters. The news spread like wildfire, and the residents of Pogsville eagerly awaited their chance to join in the slam-tastic fun.

The local news ran headlines declaring, "Pogsville's Peculiar Pog Parade: The Craziness Leaves Town in a Flurry of Flipping!"

But amidst the chaos and excitement, there were moments of sheer hilarity as the residents of Pogsville dove headfirst into the world of Pogs. Some traded their discs with fervor, while others engaged in epic battles of slammer supremacy in a comical display of competitive spirit.

But the true heroes of the day were a group of Pog enthusiasts known as the Slam Masters, who had unwittingly become the champions of Pogsville's slammer slapstick with their enthusiastic slams and strategic flips. With each flick of the wrist and each victorious shout of "Pog!", they brought joy and laughter to all who joined in the Pog pandemonium.

From that day forward, Pogsville became known as the town that had a close encounter with the Pog kind, a place where even the simplest of cardboard discs could bring people together in laughter and camaraderie.

And so, as the residents of Pogsville bid farewell to The Craziness of Pogs and continued to reminisce about their favorite slams with a smile on their faces and a stack of Pogs in their pockets, they did so knowing that they had been part of a truly hilarious and unforgettable Pog adventure.

The AIM Antics: A Hilarious Tale of Digital Dialogue

Once upon a time, in the bustling realm of Cyberspace, where pixels danced and emojis twinkled like stars in a virtual galaxy, there occurred an event that would go down in history as The Introduction of AOL Instant Messenger (AIM).

It all started with the arrival of AIM, a magical messenger that allowed people to chat with friends and family in real time, all from the comfort of their computer screens. The news spread like wildfire, and users everywhere eagerly awaited their chance to join in the digital dialogue.

The local news ran headlines declaring, "Cyberspace's Comical Chat Craze: The Introduction of AIM Leaves Town in a Sea of Smiley Faces!"

But amidst the excitement and anticipation, there were moments of sheer hilarity as users navigated the new world of instant messaging. Some fumbled with their keyboards, sending nonsensical messages in a comical display of digital dexterity, while others discovered the joy of crafting the perfect away message, filled with cryptic song lyrics or inside jokes.

But the true heroes of the day were a group of AIM aficionados known as the Chat Chatterboxes, who had unwittingly become the champions of Cyberspace's digital dialogue with their witty banter and endless stream of LOLs and ROFLs. With each "brb" and each "gtg", they brought joy and laughter to all who joined in the AIM antics.

From that day forward, Cyberspace became known as the realm that had a close encounter of the digital kind, a place where even the simplest of messages could bring people together in laughter and camaraderie.

And so, as the residents of Cyberspace bid farewell to The Introduction of AIM and continued to chat away with a smile on their faces and a keyboard at their fingertips, they did so knowing that they had been part of a truly hilarious and unforgettable digital adventure.

The Twin Peaks Whirlwind: A Zany Tale of Small-Town Mystery

Once upon a time, in the quaint town of Twin Peaks, where trees whispered secrets and owls hooted like gossiping neighbors, there occurred an event that would go down in history as The Oddity of "Twin Peaks".

It all started with the airing of a TV show called "Twin Peaks," featuring an eccentric cast of characters and a mysterious murder that rocked the sleepy town. The news spread like wildfire, and viewers everywhere eagerly tuned in to unravel the enigmatic tale.

The local news ran headlines declaring, "Twin Peaks' Peculiar Plotline: The Oddity Leaves Town in a Tizzy of Twists!"

But amidst the intrigue and suspense, there were moments of sheer hilarity as viewers watched the oddities of Twin Peaks unfold. Some scratched their heads at the cryptic clues, while others found themselves chuckling at the quirky behavior of the townsfolk in a comical display of small-town eccentricity.

But the true heroes of the day were a group of "Twin Peaks" enthusiasts known as the Peak Puzzlers, who had unwittingly become the champions of Twin Peaks' mysterious mayhem with their enthusiastic theorizing and humorous commentary. With each red herring and each plot twist, they brought joy and laughter to all who joined in the Twin Peaks whirlwind.

From that day forward, Twin Peaks became known as the town that had a close encounter of the mystery kind, a place where even the strangest of occurrences could bring people together in laughter and camaraderie.

And so, as the residents of Twin Peaks bid farewell to The Oddity of "Twin Peaks" and continued to ponder the mysteries of their beloved town with a smile on their faces and a twinkle in their eyes, they did so knowing that they had been part of a truly hilarious and unforgettable small-town adventure.

The Grunge Fashion Frenzy: A Wacky Tale of Flannel and Doc Martens

Once upon a time, in the bustling streets of Trendsville, where fashionistas strutted and designers schemed like couture kings and queens, there occurred an event that would go down in history as The Rise of Grunge Fashion.

It all started with the emergence of grunge, a rebellious style that celebrated flannel shirts, ripped jeans, and combat boots. The news spread like wildfire, and fashionistas everywhere eagerly embraced the laid-back look of the Pacific Northwest.

The local news ran headlines declaring, "Trendsville's Tumultuous Trend Tornado: The Rise of Grunge Fashion Leaves Town in a Plaid Pandemonium!"

But amidst the chaos and confusion, there were moments of sheer hilarity as the residents of Trendsville attempted to master the art of grunge fashion. Some raided their parents' closets for old flannels, while others tried to distress their jeans with questionable results in a comical display of DIY disasters.

But the true heroes of the day were a group of grunge enthusiasts known as the Flannel Fanatics, who had unwittingly become the champions of Trendsville's grunge revolution with their unkempt hair and devil-may-care attitude. With each plaid-clad ensemble and each stomping step in their Doc Martens, they brought joy and laughter to all who joined in the grunge fashion frenzy.

From that day forward, Trendsville became known as the town that had a close encounter of the grunge kind, a place where even the most mismatched of outfits could bring people together in laughter and camaraderie.

And so, as the residents of Trendsville bid farewell to The Rise of Grunge Fashion and continued to embrace their newfound style with a smile on their faces and a guitar riff in their hearts, they did so knowing that they had been part of a truly hilarious and unforgettable fashion adventure.

The Simpsons Shenanigans: A Zany Tale of Yellow Family Hijinks

Once upon a time, in the colorful town of Springfield, where donuts rolled and nuclear power plants hummed like symphonies of chaos, there occurred an event that would go down in history as The Absurdity of "The Simpsons".

It all started with the debut of a TV show called "The Simpsons," featuring a family of yellow-skinned misfits and their quirky adventures. The news spread like wildfire, and viewers everywhere eagerly tuned in to join the hilarity-filled escapades.

The local news ran headlines declaring, "Springfield's Spectacular Simpson Shenanigans: The Absurdity Leaves Town in Stitches!"

But amidst the laughter and chaos, there were moments of sheer hilarity as viewers watched the antics of Homer, Marge, Bart, Lisa, and Maggie unfold. Some shook their heads at Homer's bumbling antics, while others found themselves in stitches at Bart's mischievous pranks in a comical display of animated absurdity.

But the true heroes of the day were a group of "The Simpsons" enthusiasts known as the Springfield Sillies, who had unwittingly become the champions of Springfield's cartoon chaos with their enthusiastic discussions and humorous impressions. With each "D'oh!" and each "Ay caramba!", they brought joy and laughter to all who joined in the Simpson shenanigans.

From that day forward, Springfield became known as the town that had a close encounter of the animated kind, a place where even the most absurd of situations could bring people together in laughter and camaraderie.

And so, as the residents of Springfield bid farewell to The Absurdity of "The Simpsons" and continued to enjoy their favorite episodes with a smile on their faces and a chuckle in their hearts, they did so knowing that they had been part of a truly hilarious and unforgettable animated adventure.

The O.J. Simpson Saga: A Quirky Tale of Courtroom Capers

Once upon a time, in the bustling courtroom of Los Angeles, where gavels banged and reporters scribbled like mad, there occurred an event that would go down in history as The Oddity of the O.J. Simpson Trial.

It all started with the trial of O.J. Simpson, a former football star accused of a double murder. The news spread like wildfire, and people across the nation were glued to their TVs, eagerly awaiting each twist and turn in the courtroom drama.

The local news ran headlines declaring, "Los Angeles' Lively Legal Limelight: The Oddity of the O.J. Simpson Trial Leaves Town in a Tizzy!"

But amidst the drama and intrigue, there were moments of sheer hilarity as spectators watched the proceedings unfold. Some marveled at the bizarre antics of the defense team, while others found themselves in stitches at the antics of the courtroom characters in a comical display of legal lunacy.

But the true heroes of the day were a group of trial enthusiasts known as the Courtroom Comedians, who had unwittingly become the champions of Los Angeles' legal lunacy with their witty commentary and humorous observations. With each eyebrow raised and each whispered aside, they brought joy and laughter to all who joined in the O.J. Simpson saga.

From that day forward, Los Angeles became known as the city that had a close encounter of the courtroom kind, a place where even the most serious of trials could bring people together in laughter and camaraderie.

And so, as the residents of Los Angeles bid farewell to The Oddity of the O.J. Simpson Trial and continued to reflect on the trial with a smile on their faces and a chuckle in their hearts, they did so knowing that they had been part of a truly hilarious and unforgettable legal adventure.

The Dial-Up Delight: A Hilarious Journey into the World Wide Web

Once upon a time, in the not-so-distant past, there was a magical era known as the age of dial-up internet. It was a time when the internet was a mysterious and wondrous place, accessed through the magical tones of a dial-up modem.

In every town and city, families gathered around their bulky desktop computers, eagerly awaiting the screeching sound of the modem connecting to the World Wide Web. It was a moment of anticipation and excitement, as if embarking on a digital adventure.

The local news ran headlines declaring, "The Dial-Up Delight: The Quirky Quest for Internet Access Leaves Town in a Tangle of Wires!"

But amidst the excitement, there were moments of sheer hilarity as users navigated the quirks of dial-up internet. Some waited patiently as web pages loaded at a snail's pace, while others endured the frustration of being disconnected mid-surf in a comical display of technological woes.

But the true heroes of the day were a group of internet enthusiasts known as the Cyber Surfers, who had unwittingly become the champions of the dial-up era with their persistence and determination to explore the vast reaches of the internet. With each painstakingly slow download and each dropped connection, they brought joy and laughter to all who joined in the dial-up delight.

From that day forward, the era of dial-up internet became known as a time of digital discovery and technological triumph, a period where even the most mundane of internet tasks could bring people together in laughter and camaraderie.

And so, as the residents of towns and cities bid farewell to The Dial-Up Delight and embraced the lightning-fast speeds of broadband internet, they did so with a fondness for the quirky era that had brought them so much laughter and joy.

The Seinfeld Saga: A Hilarious Romp Through Sitcom Shenanigans

Once upon a time, in the bustling city of New York, where taxis honked and pigeons strutted like extras in a sitcom set, there occurred an event that would go down in history as The Hilarity of "Seinfeld".

It all started with the debut of a TV show called "Seinfeld," featuring a group of friends and their absurd misadventures in everyday life. The news spread like wildfire, and viewers everywhere eagerly tuned in to join the laughter-filled escapades.

The local news ran headlines declaring, "New York's Nonsensical 'Seinfeld' Shenanigans: The Hilarity Leaves Town in Stitches!"

But amidst the laughter and absurdity, there were moments of sheer hilarity as viewers watched the antics of Jerry, George, Elaine, and

Kramer unfold. Some shook their heads at Jerry's neuroticism, while others found themselves in stitches at Kramer's wacky schemes in a comical display of sitcom silliness.

But the true heroes of the day were a group of "Seinfeld" enthusiasts known as the Sitcom Sages, who had unwittingly become the champions of New York's sitcom shenanigans with their enthusiastic recitations of iconic lines and spot-on impressions. With each "yada yada" and each "No soup for you!", they brought joy and laughter to all who joined in the "Seinfeld" saga.

From that day forward, New York became known as the city that had a close encounter of the sitcom kind, a place where even the most mundane of situations could bring people together in laughter and camaraderie.

And so, as the residents of New York bid farewell to The Hilarity of "Seinfeld" and continued to rewatch their favorite episodes with a smile on their faces and a chuckle in their hearts, they did so knowing that they had been part of a truly hilarious and unforgettable sitcom adventure.

www.ingramcontent.com/pod-product-compliance
Lightning Source LLC
Chambersburg PA
CBHW081157020426
42333CB00020B/2533